First Class Delivery

1 Women's Experiences and Opinions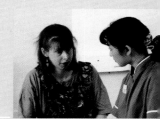

2 Care of Women in Pregnancy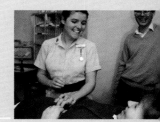

3 Care of Women in Labour and Birth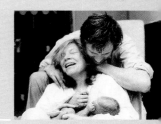

4 Care of Women after Childbirth and the Care of Newborn Babies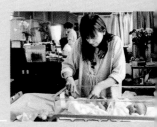

5 The Way Forward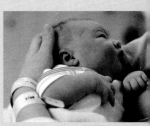

Contents

Preface		**3**
Introduction		**4**
Structure of the report		7
1	**Women's Experiences and Opinions**	**9**
	Women's perceptions and attitudes	11
	Choice and information	13
	Continuity of care	15
	Conclusions	16
2	**Care of Women in Pregnancy**	**17**
	Introduction	18
	The organisation of antenatal care	21
	Number of antenatal checks	25
	Clinical content of antenatal checks	27
	Recommendations	30
3	**Care of Women in Labour and Birth**	**32**
	Introduction	33
	Caring for women in labour	35
	Midwife staffing	37
	Medical interventions – providing effective care	41
	Recommendations	48

4	**Care of Women after Childbirth and the Care of Newborn Babies**	**50**
	Introduction	51
	Efficient postnatal care	52
	The quality of postnatal care	57
	Care of sick babies in neonatal units	58
	Recommendations	65
5	**The Way Forward**	**67**
	Introduction	68
	Variations in patterns of care	68
	Fragmentation	69
	Women-centred services: information and choice	70
	Improving efficiency	71
	Effective care	72
	Conclusions	72
	Recommendations	73

Appendix 1: Data Sources and Research Methods	**74**
Appendix 2: Advisory Group and Other Advisers	**82**
Abbreviations	**84**
Glossary	**85**
References	**88**
Bibliography	**94**
Index	**97**

© Audit Commission 1997

First published in March 1997 by the Audit Commission for Local Authorities and the National Health Service in England and Wales, 1 Vincent Square, London SW1P 2PN

Printed in the UK for the Audit Commission by Kent Litho

ISBN 1 86240 023 7

Photography:
Pictor International (cover, p3, p5, p67); Lupe Cunha Photography (p9, p17); Sally & Richard Greenhill (p14, p29, p32, p42, p50, p78); Maggie Murray/Format (p18); Sue de Jong/Format (p37).

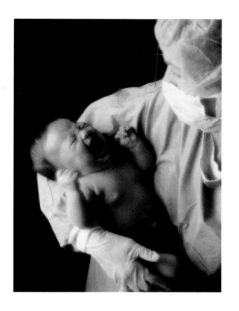

Preface

The Audit Commission oversees the external audit of the National Health Service (NHS) and local authorities in England and Wales. As part of this function, the Commission is required to carry out studies to enable it to make recommendations for improving the economy, efficiency and effectiveness of services provided by these bodies.

Over the last two years, the Commission has reviewed maternity services in the NHS, which take care of 650,000 women and their babies each year. This study collected information from 13 NHS trusts that provide both hospital and community-based maternity care, 2,375 recent mothers, 12 commissioning authorities and 300 GPs (See Appendix 1 for details of data sources). This report sets out the findings of this work.

The report is aimed mainly at managers and purchasers of maternity services. It reviews the extent and direction of the changes that are occurring in response to policy, and attempts to identify how progress can be achieved.

The Commission's auditors will undertake local audits of maternity services at every trust in England and Wales during 1997. The large scale of the service, the widely varying levels of resource use and the organisational change which is currently taking place make the Audit Commission review particularly timely. Maternity services have been high on the agenda of both purchasers and providers, and this report will add an important focus on efficiency and the cost of services.

The study on which this report is based was carried out by Beverley Fitzsimons, Jane Laughton, John Bailey and Emma Windred within the Health Studies Directorate of the Commission, and Maggie Redshaw of the Institute of Child Health, University of Bristol, under the direction of Jocelyn Cornwell and Jonathan Boyce. Statistical support was provided by Jo Marsh, Maire O'Sullivan, Lara Bryant, Mark Pilling and Salima Nanji, and administrative support by Angela Lane. The team was advised by a group of experts listed at Appendix 2.

'Maternity services are very popular with women and their families, and compare favourably in this respect with most other NHS services.'

Introduction

1. For the past few years there has been considerable debate about maternity care, as evidenced in the number of government and other reports and publications (Refs. 1–5). In England, maternity services are high on the management agenda as health authorities and trusts reach the mid-point of a timetable set by the Government for implementing the recommendations in *Changing Childbirth* (Ref. 5). Wales has its own policy (Ref. 4). This report, and the associated local audits in NHS trusts in England and Wales, aims to help those who run maternity services to maximise the benefit they can obtain from available resources while responding positively to the policy emphasis on centring services more on women.

2. Maternity services provide care for women in pregnancy, during labour and childbirth and care for mothers and babies postnatally. They are provided by a range of professions in primary, community and secondary care settings at a gross cost of £1.1billion or around £1,700 per delivery (Ref. 6).

3. The foundation for the organisation of services was laid when mortality and morbidity for mothers and babies were high and there was concern about poor living conditions. In the intervening years there have been two parallel developments: maternal and perinatal mortality and morbidity have declined, particularly from the middle of the century, and maternity care has become increasingly medical- and hospital-based. As these outcomes have improved, the trend towards almost universal hospital births has given credence to the widely held view that pregnancy and birth are inherently dangerous and risky and can be regarded as normal only after the event.

4. Maternity services are very popular with women and their families, and compare favourably in this respect with most other NHS services. They are different from other health services in a number of important ways. Firstly, women who use the service are not like other 'patients'. They are generally well, and often hold firm views about how their care should be provided. Through the National Childbirth Trust and other campaigning consumer groups, their influence has been considerable. Most campaigns have been about giving women more say over their care, more information about the options available to them and more choice. Their success is due in part to the fact that their arguments are supported by scientific research that demonstrates that emotional and psychological aspects of care affect outcomes for mothers (Ref. 7).

5. Secondly, unlike other areas, there are differing views about what services are for. While all involved agree that the well-being of the mother and baby are paramount, there are two schools of thought about how this might best be achieved. One group believes that, because of the inherent risks and complications associated with childbearing, medical surveillance should be promoted for all women. Others believe that, while this should be available for those women who need or choose it, the majority of women would benefit from a service that supported and cared for them without medical involvement during what is most often an uncomplicated and safe event. This division (which is not between professional and lay points of view – there are equally committed obstetricians, midwives, GPs and service users in both camps) polarises discussion and debates about service strategy and priorities.

6. Thirdly, obstetrics and paediatrics were among the first medical specialties to look for evidence of clinical effectiveness, and to establish a tradition of systematic reviews of maternal deaths, stillbirths and deaths in infancy (CEMD and CESDI) (Refs. 8, 9). More recently, the Cochrane database of clinical trials has broadened the definitions applied to outcomes of care and offered clinicians a wider grasp of maternity-related research (Ref. 10).

7. The policy agenda for maternity care prioritises 'woman-centred' services (Refs. 4, 5). It identifies efficiency and effectiveness as service objectives but emphasises information, choice, continuity of carer, flexibility and listening to women's views (Box A, overleaf). In Wales, the policy gives equal weight to the objectives of clinical effectiveness, efficient use of resources and strengthening the focus on service users (Refs. 4, 11). Both policies were well received by professional and consumer groups and provided a welcome impetus for change.

8. Clinical staff and managers of maternity services can rightly be proud of the service for which they are responsible. Women are on the whole pleased with their care and staff are well motivated and positive about the services that they provide. Around three-quarters of the staff surveyed by the Commission believe that the way services are organised is good for women and nine out of ten agree that they gain great job satisfaction from their work. But the service faces important challenges and there is concern about the degree to which expanding the range of options and giving women more choice is compatible with efficient service delivery within finite resources.

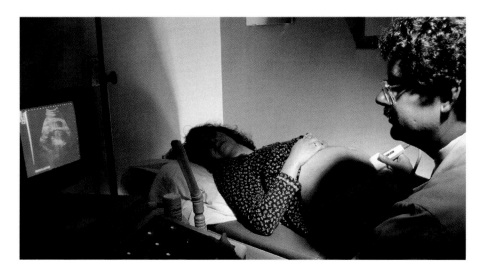

Box A
Policies for maternity services in England and Wales

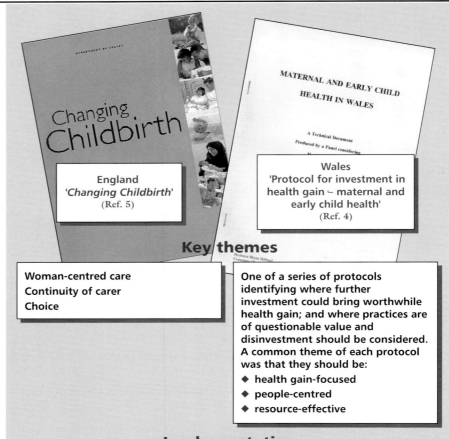

England
'*Changing Childbirth*'
(Ref. 5)

Wales
'Protocol for investment in health gain – maternal and early child health'
(Ref. 4)

Key themes

Woman-centred care
Continuity of carer
Choice

One of a series of protocols identifying where further investment could bring worthwhile health gain; and where practices are of questionable value and disinvestment should be considered. A common theme of each protocol was that they should be:

◆ health gain-focused
◆ people-centred
◆ resource-effective

Implementation

Purchasers instructed through NHS Priorities and Planning Guidance to:

◆ ask women what they want
◆ ensure services have local women's support
◆ deliver efficient and effective services with good clinical outcomes

Purchasers and providers are directed to aim for a woman-centred service as defined by ten 'indicators of success' with:

◆ an increasing role for the midwife (*Changing Childbirth* indicators 3, 6, 7)
◆ more continuity of care (*Changing Childbirth* indicators 1, 2, 4, 5)
◆ better information (*Changing Childbirth* indicators 1, 10)

Purchasers and providers have targets set for health gain, the quality of childbirth and early childhood for both mother and child and resource use. They include:

◆ reductions in childhood deaths and morbidity
◆ reductions in births of children with unexpected handicaps
◆ women to have more informed choice
◆ better measurement of consumer satisfaction
◆ better research into women's preferences
◆ better targeting of resources towards women in need of specialist care and away from women with uncomplicated pregnancies

9. Bringing about simultaneous improvements in quality of service to the user, and in efficiency and clinical effectiveness, puts midwives, obstetricians and managers under considerable pressure. This report has identified a number of important concerns:

- There is wide variation in the sort of service offered that cannot be attributed to women's own choices about the care that they would like. There is considerable emphasis at present on providing individualised and personalised services, but many women report having limited choice and control over key aspects of their care and say that they lack information (see Chapter 1).

- For some women, maternity care is fragmented between a number of providers – either different trusts, or trusts and GPs, who may not be delivering continuity of care. And sometimes care provided by a single trust lacks continuity.

- The use of resources in maternity services varies considerably from place to place (Exhibit 1, overleaf) – differences that cannot be linked to indicators of need. In addition, it is not always as efficient as it could be, for example in the balance that is struck between the care provided in hospital and in the community.

- In some areas of care, services are out of step with the current consensus on good practice. In others, purchasers and trusts are hampered by a lack of clear evidence about what is the best way to provide a clinically effective service. This is particularly true of postnatal care.

- Other changes in the broader NHS, such as the changes in junior doctors' training and reductions in their hours, are having a direct impact on the service. Looking ahead, there may be new developments in primary care maternity provision (Ref. 12) and GPs, regardless of fundholding status, are likely to become more involved in determining local service strategies.

Structure of the report

10. The first chapter of this report presents the findings from an Audit Commission survey that asked a a nationally representative sample of recent mothers about their experience and views of maternity care (see Appendix 1 for details of the survey methodology; the survey findings will be published in full in a separate report). We ask whether, and in what respects, women feel maternity services are responsive to their needs, focusing on those aspects of services highlighted in *Changing Childbirth*.

11. The chapters that follow examine the phases of maternity care from three different perspectives: women's view of their care; efficiency of service provision; and effectiveness in clinical practice. Throughout, the report treats the three perspectives as equally important. Chapter 2 is about care in pregnancy; Chapter 3 about care in labour and delivery, and Chapter 4 about postnatal care in hospital and at home. Chapter 4 also looks at the care of babies in neonatal units.

12. The final chapter revisits the main themes of the report and makes recommendations to purchasers and trusts that will help them take services forward into the 21st century.

Exhibit 1
Numbers of deliveries per consultant and midwife at NHS trusts

The mix of staff in maternity care varies considerably between trusts.

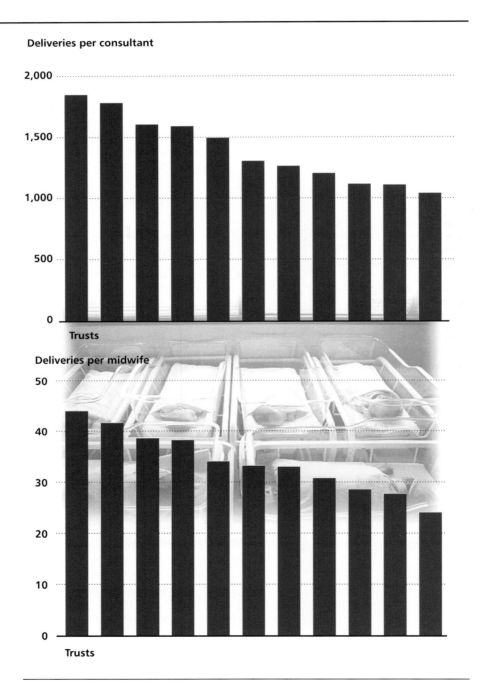

Deliveries per consultant

Trusts

Deliveries per midwife

Trusts

Note: Data on consultants is for obstetrics only. Where obstetrics and gynaecology are combined, 50 per cent is used. Trusts are all non-teaching.

Source: Audit Commission study sites

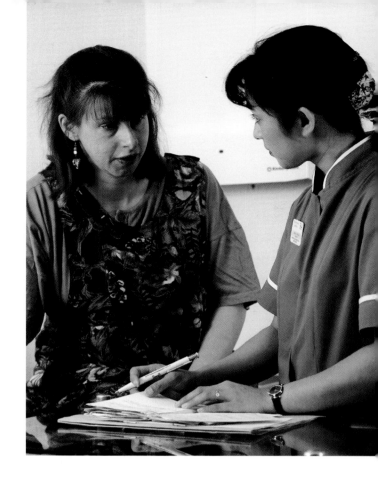

1 Women's Experiences and Opinions

Maternity services place a high priority on the satisfaction of women and their families. On the whole, women rate them highly.

However, some groups of women have less positive experiences, and some aspects of care – most particularly postnatal care – are generally less satisfactory. To women using the services, interpersonal and emotional, as well as clinical aspects of care, are important.

Given the widescale reorganisation of services currently taking place, purchasers and trusts should take the views of local service users into account when they are setting service priorities.

13. 'Patients and their families hold unique vantage points as expert witnesses to care' (Ref. 13). Health professionals increasingly recognise the value of information that can be obtained from service users. Similarly, purchasers and managers find that information from users can help them with difficult decisions about providing local services.

14. Women rate maternity services very highly and the services give high priority to the satisfaction of women and their families. However, some women have a poor experience, (either clinically or in their personal care) and the recollection of this remains for many years, affecting their sense of themselves, their recollection of the experience and their attitude to future pregnancies (Refs. 14, 15).

15. Safety is always a prime concern to women, their families and professionals. But the distinctive nature of the service – providing care and support for a predominantly healthy population through a normal life event, the policy emphasis on woman-centred care, and the impact of women's subjective experiences of care on outcomes, have also brought other issues centre stage. This chapter examines women's perceptions of, and attitudes towards, maternity care and asks, to what extent the service is achieving a more user-centred focus? It draws upon an Audit Commission survey of recent mothers (Box B) as well as other published sources, and concentrates, in particular, on three indicators of quality of care (emphasised in current maternity policies): choice, information and continuity of care (Refs. 4, 5).

Box B
Audit Commission survey of recent mothers

Scope and purpose	To obtain information about current patterns of maternity care
	To investigate women's opinions of aspects of their care
	To provide information on issues of current concern in policy, namely: choice, information and continuity of care
Method	Retrospective postal questionnaire based on methods by Mason et al (Ref. 16). Piloting and subsequent administration carried out by MORI health research group in Nov – Dec 1995
Sample	Random sample of 3,570 women four months postnatally drawn by OPCS from births registers of all registration districts of England and Wales
	Overall response rate of 67 per cent (2,375 women)
	983 women also volunteered comments about aspects of their care (see Appendix 1)
Respondent profile	Respondents broadly representative in terms of age and region
	Over-represents women from social classes I and II (52 per cent vs. 45 per cent of original sample)
	Under-represents women with no educational qualifications (12 per cent vs. 20 per cent in original sample)

Note: See tables 6-10 in Appendix 1 for details of the respondents to the survey.

Source: Audit Commission

Women's perceptions and attitudes

16. The vast majority of women rate maternity care very positively (Exhibit 2). But the feelings of gratitude and relief that naturally predominate in relation to childbirth make it important to develop specific and sensitive research methods that can get behind responses to general questions about satisfaction with services, to find out in detail what happens to mothers and how they feel about their care (Refs. 17, 18). If women are asked about specific aspects of the service and if they are able to volunteer information about their care, they can help to identify areas that should be targeted for improvement.

Exhibit 2
Women's perceptions of different aspects of maternity care

Most women are pleased with their maternity care overall.

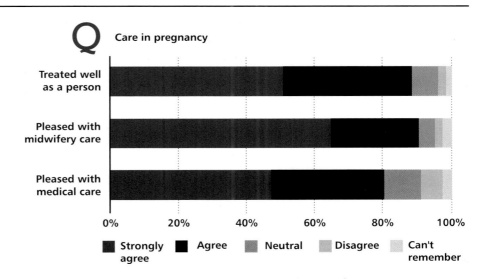

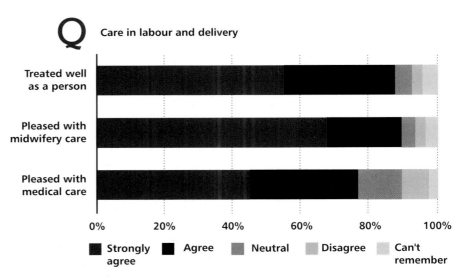

Source: Audit Commission survey of recent mothers (N = 2,375)

'Women are more satisfied with the clinical than with the inter-personal and emotional aspects of care.'

17. Some aspects of maternity care matter to women more than others. The large number of 'free text' comments they spontaneously made on questionnaires about emotional support (314 comments) and the quality of medical and midwifery care (473 comments) indicate that both are especially important. Women are more satisfied with the clinical than with the inter-personal and emotional aspects of care. Dissatisfaction with inter-personal aspects of care is particularly important, given their influence on outcomes. Two-thirds of the comments about clinical aspects of care were positive as compared with less than one-third of the comments about inter-personal factors (Appendix 1, Table 10) .

18. The message from the survey for purchasers and NHS trusts is that women have very different experiences, expectations and views. A variety of factors are important, including age and social background, whether it is a first pregnancy or a pregnancy with complications, and the way that services are organised. Women's expectations of the service and sense of control over the experience also matter (Refs. 17, 18).

19. Particular subgroups are significantly less satisfied with some aspects of care. Women having their first baby and those who are younger are significantly less likely than other mothers to say that they had all the support and information that they needed in labour, and more likely to say that they saw too many different staff. Older women are more likely to be confident and are more satisfied with their communication with health professionals than younger women. Those from minority ethnic groups are less likely to report feeling that they were treated with respect and kindness. And women with more complex needs in pregnancy are less likely than others to respond positively to questions about their care.

20. Women's views about aspects such as where and by whom care is provided vary according to the phase of care. During pregnancy, many prefer local, community-based care. Recent studies suggest that this is preferred because they find it more personal and more informative than the care they receive in hospital (Ref. 19). In the Commission's survey, women who had 'shared' antenatal care – that is, whose antenatal checks took place both in hospital and in the community – preferred the community-based elements of their care (Exhibit 3). The reasons for their preference – whether it is the location itself, the less busy environment, the smaller number of professionals, or other factors that make community-based clinics more popular – are not clear.

21. In labour and birth, women who have difficult deliveries or medical problems feel less positive about their experience than other women. This is perhaps inevitable, but researchers have found that the effects of such difficult experiences can be reduced if services are organised appropriately (for example, Ref. 19) with women feeling greater confidence and having a better understanding of birth events.

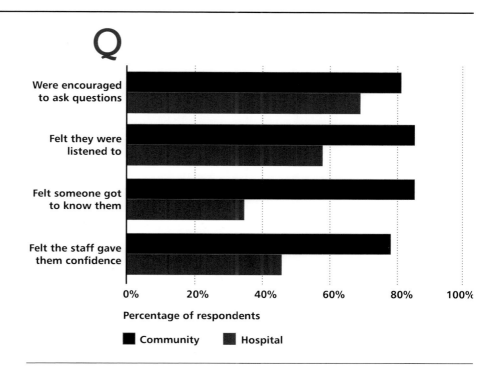

Exhibit 3
Women's perceptions of hospital and community-based care in pregnancy

Women who had 'shared' antenatal care preferred the community-based elements.

Note: All differences are significant.
p = <0.001

Source: Audit Commission survey of recent mothers (N = 1,200 women identified as receiving shared care)

22. Postnatally, hospital care was the subject of particularly critical comment in the Commission's survey, a finding which is echoed elsewhere (Ref. 19). Issues such as staffing levels, facilities, food, and cleanliness and hygiene are frequently mentioned and availability of support from staff is of particular concern. This contrasts with women's views of postnatal care at home, which is highly popular.

Choice and information

23. Women clearly value good communication with the professionals looking after them. Information is important in itself and is part of enabling women to make choices and feel involved in their care. The extent to which professionals are succeeding in giving women as much information as they want varies partly by subject matter, partly by service. It is important to be able to ask questions and be listened to, and women often find this easier in community clinics than in hospital.

24. The Commission asked women about two aspects of choice: the degree to which they felt they were offered a range of options for care; and the extent to which they felt their own wishes had been taken into account in reaching decisions.

25. Only one in three women felt that they definitely had a say in where they went for antenatal care and who provided it. Over half of the women to whom it applied, however, felt fully involved in the more specific decisions that were made about whether they should have particular screening tests and scans.

26. In labour and delivery, where it is especially important that women feel in control of what happens to them, the sense of involvement in the decisions that are taken varies between individuals and procedures (see Chapter 3, Exhibit 11). These procedures include the way in which the baby was monitored in labour, whether to start or speed up labour, and whether to perform an episiotomy. For example, while one in five women felt that they had a full say in how their baby was monitored, at the opposite extreme, more than half felt that they had no say at all. Providing good information and the opportunity for discussion is likely to reduce women's disappointment when their experiences do not match their hopes and expectations.

27. Postnatally, women for the most part say that the length of their hospital stay, and the frequency of visits by the community midwife to them at home, were about right (72 per cent and 80 per cent). But roughly one-quarter of women felt that the service could have met their needs better. Involving women in discussions about the most appropriate time to go home is particularly important, with women who felt that they had a say in the decision about their length of stay nearly twice as likely to feel that the service was right for them. Information in the form of a debriefing facility is also valued by many women (Refs. 20, 21).

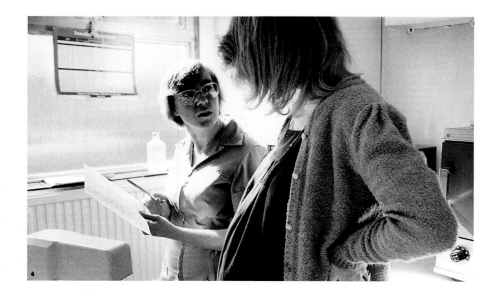

Continuity of care

28. Continuity of care (which means that care is delivered in a consistent way, regardless of the professional providing it) is important to all women. Continuity of carer, on the other hand, means that care is provided by a small number of professionals, or by professionals whom women know. Moreover, it is important only to some women. Although it is not clear what it is about 'continuity' which is of particular benefit, evidence shows that women are less likely to feel satisfied with their care if they consider it to be fragmented.

29. Some trusts have decided that continuity of carer within labour is most important and try to provide continuous support by the same midwife throughout labour. Just over 80 per cent of women in the survey felt that this was important, although only half said that their care was provided this way. In practice, some women see many different faces during labour: one in three in the survey were looked after by three or more midwives at different times in labour. In some cases, more staff are involved because the labour is especially long or complicated, but in others the lack of continuity is caused by the approach taken to staffing the labour ward.

30. Other trusts have decided to promote greater continuity across antenatal care, labour and delivery and postnatal care, and have experimented with different ways of organising midwives. Some have established team midwifery with small teams of midwives providing all the midwifery care (antenatal, in labour and postnatal care) to women on their caseload. This limits the number of different midwives involved in caring for the same individual, and theoretically at least, women and midwives get to know one another and women will know at least some of the professionals who look after them in labour. Just over half the women in the Commission's survey felt that it was important to meet the staff before labour begins, and they were more likely to hold this view if that had been their actual experience.

31. In postnatal hospital care, women value the opportunity to discuss their care with someone they know and who knows what happened during their labour. Women who had this opportunity feel more confident and more satisfied with their care. Postnatal home visits by midwives are highly valued by most women, regardless of whether they had met the midwives before. However, the potential disruption to continuity of carer, with 40 per cent of women seeing three or more different midwives during the postnatal period, may be a useful focus for providers, given the long-cited problem of conflicting advice (for example, Ref. 22).

32. It is clear that continuity of carer is important for some women, but it is not clear which is the best way of providing this, or whether it is always the top priority. Reorganising services to provide continuity of carer across phases of care can have resource implications. This means that trusts and purchasers must work out the relative importance that different groups and subgroups attach to particular features of services before they start to make changes.

'Continuity of care... is important to all women. Continuity of carer, on the other hand... is important only to some.'

Conclusions

33. Most women rate their maternity care very highly overall, but some women have a poor experience, and some aspects of care can be the focus of particular criticism: it is this diversity that presents a particular challenge for providing woman-centred care. Asking service users their views of services can help to identify priorities for change, and is particularly useful since the information obtained crosses professional boundaries. For example, surveys have identified women's concerns about duplication of antenatal services, with 'booking visits' being repeated in the hospital and the community; their concerns about being left alone in labour have helped managers to focus on arrangements for staffing labour wards; and, postnatally, conflicting policies and practices about breastfeeding have also been successfully highlighted using user surveys.

34. The methods in use for gathering information from service users are still developing: data can vary according to how, when and by whom questions are asked, and satisfaction indices can be confounded by expectations of services and service outcomes. This does not mean that evidence from users is not valid: it can be used with care to provide guidance on opportunities for service improvements. Different methods may be needed to involve different groups of women, such as non English-speakers. Maternity Services Liaison Committees (MSLCs) can also be a valuable means of involving local women in decision-making.

35. The Audit Commission survey suggests some areas where improvements are clearly possible in the way in which services are delivered. In particular, there is substantial dissatisfaction with the information that women receive. This is important in itself, and also because it affects other aspects of care, such as whether women feel that they have choices and options.

36. It is important to focus services on the needs of women, and it is essential that these needs are identified by asking women themselves before decisions are made to change the service. Changing the organisation of the service may raise already high expectations: more of those women who are offered, for example, continuity of carer across phases of care, will go on to rate this as an important aspect of the service than those who are not offered it. For these reasons, it is vital that any decisions to make changes are firmly based on evidence, especially given the number of competing priorities for action.

37. Survey data can help to identify priorities. But effectiveness and efficiency issues need to be considered alongside women's views of care. The following chapters review each of these issues for each phase of maternity care.

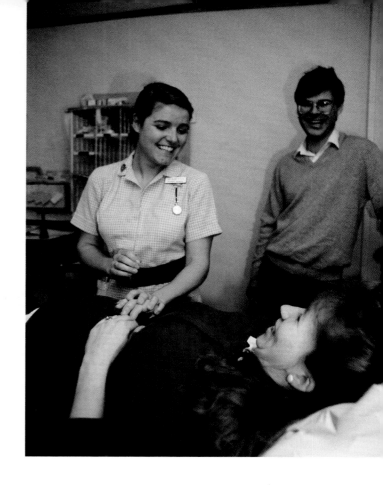

2 Care of Women in Pregnancy

Current policy emphasises the importance of women's choice in relation to all aspects of antenatal care. In practice, women feel that they have less say over some aspects of care than others and substantial numbers would like to have more information about their options for care and services. Information is particularly important in antenatal screening, where the tests themselves have the potential to cause great anxiety.

The extent to which obstetricians routinely see women with uncomplicated pregnancies varies. Trusts should aim to base the care of these women in the community, with care provided by midwives and GPs. Not only does community care cost significantly less than traditional, obstetrician-led, shared care, but it is more appropriate and probably more satisfactory for many of these women.

Trusts should develop antenatal care policies which take account of women's needs for information, support and reassurance, and review the number of checks that they offer to women. They will need to define clinical objectives and the timing and frequency of the activities needed to achieve them.

Introduction

38. Antenatal care is needed to monitor the health of women and their babies and to treat identified problems; to provide information, support and reassurance; and to screen for specific fetal abnormalities.

39. Care during pregnancy is provided at antenatal check-ups by midwives, GPs and hospital doctors, either singly or in combination. It takes place in the community in GPs' surgeries and occasionally in the woman's home; in the hospital setting, and often in some combination of these settings (Exhibit 4). Some women also stay in hospital antenatally, and some spend time in antenatal day assessment facilities.

40. It is current policy to give women as much choice as possible over aspects of their antenatal care, such as where they will be seen, which professionals will undertake their care, and which services they will be offered. They need information to take part in the discussions with professionals about these decisions. In practice, however, women feel that they have more say over some aspects of care than others (Exhibit 5) and substantial numbers express dissatisfaction with the information that they are given (Exhibit 6, overleaf).

41. The remainder of this chapter is about the main elements of antenatal care for which there is reliable guidance on efficiency and effectiveness of services – the organisation of antenatal care (where it takes place and who provides it), the number of antenatal checks that women receive, and what they comprise.

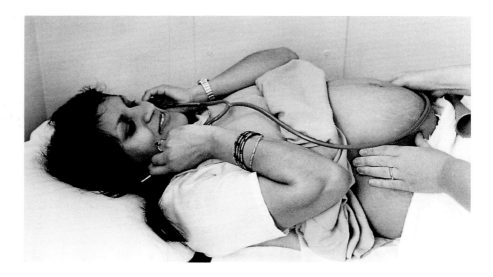

Exhibit 4
Patterns of antenatal care

Women can have antenatal checks in hospital, in the local community or in a combination of both settings.

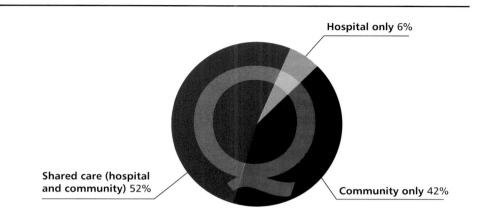

Hospital only 6%

Shared care (hospital and community) 52%

Community only 42%

Source: Audit Commission survey of recent mothers (N= 2,299)

Exhibit 5
Perceived options in antenatal care

Women feel that they have more say over some aspects of care than others.

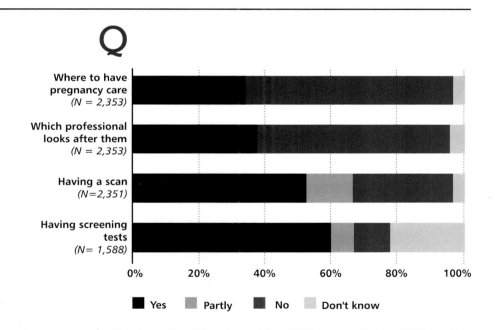

Source: Audit Commission survey of recent mothers

First Class Delivery
Improving Maternity Services in England and Wales

Exhibit 6
Women's assessment of information and communication in antenatal care

Substantial numbers of women are not satisfied with the information that they receive.

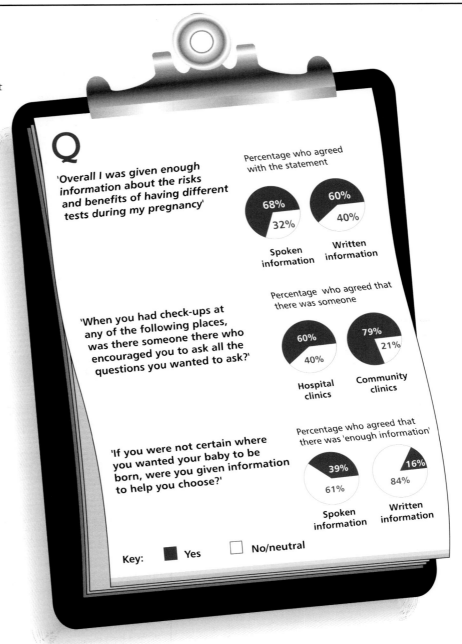

Q

'Overall I was given enough information about the risks and benefits of having different tests during my pregnancy'

Percentage who agreed with the statement

68% / 32%
Spoken information

60% / 40%
Written information

'When you had check-ups at any of the following places, was there someone there who encouraged you to ask all the questions you wanted to ask?'

Percentage who agreed that there was someone

60% / 40%
Hospital clinics

79% / 21%
Community clinics

'If you were not certain where you wanted your baby to be born, were you given information to help you choose?'

Percentage who agreed that there was 'enough information'

39% / 61%
Spoken information

16% / 84%
Written information

Key: ■ Yes   ☐ No/neutral

Source: Audit Commission survey of recent mothers

The organisation of antenatal care

42. Most women who discover that they are pregnant go to their local general practice. They usually make initial contact for antenatal care in the first 12 weeks of pregnancy (89 per cent in the Audit Commission survey, rising to 96 per cent by 16 weeks). Seventy-five per cent see a GP and most of the rest see a midwife. What happens next depends on the GP, midwife or local consultant's usual practice, on the woman's health and obstetric history and her preferences, and on the prevailing pattern of care in that locality. The GP or midwife may make the decision about what antenatal care is required, or they may refer the woman to a consultant clinic where a consultant obstetrician (or a member of their team) will decide on the most appropriate pattern of antenatal care to be provided (Exhibit 7). Care during the remainder of pregnancy is provided in various ways. It may take place entirely in the practice, provided by the GP, the midwife, or both; or it may take place entirely in hospital clinics, by hospital doctors and midwives. Some women attend antenatal clinics in both settings (in various proportions), and a minority receive care from midwives in community health centres (other than GP practices) or in their own homes.

Exhibit 7
Arrangements for making decisions about pregnancy care

The way that decisions about antenatal care are taken varies, depending on the individual woman and local policies.

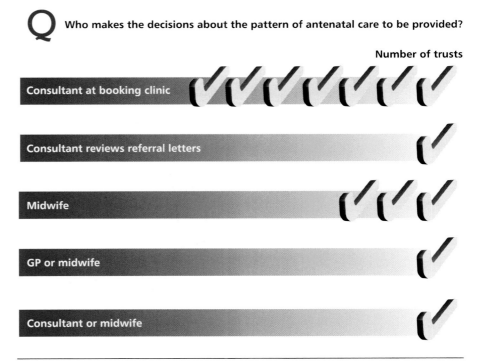

Q **Who makes the decisions about the pattern of antenatal care to be provided?**

Number of trusts

Consultant at booking clinic

Consultant reviews referral letters

Midwife

GP or midwife

Consultant or midwife

Source: Audit Commission study sites

'...patterns of antenatal care... determine the amount of choice and continuity of care available, and have cost implications.'

43. Trusts and individual consultant obstetricians differ in the extent to which they routinely provide medical input to the care of women with uncomplicated pregnancies, ranging from no consultant input, to four or more routine contacts. Obstetricians are specialists: yet in some trusts they routinely see women with uncomplicated pregnancies when community-based maternity care, provided by midwives and GPs, would be more appropriate and probably more satisfactory for many of these women. Reports from GPs confirm the varying levels of medical input for women with uncomplicated pregnancies who attend hospital clinics, with 19 per cent reporting that the referred women had no routine contact with hospital doctors, 20 per cent one contact, 39 per cent two contacts, and 21 per cent three or more. Despite this variation, the vast majority of GPs surveyed (86 per cent) felt that the level of specialist input was 'just right'.

44. The extent to which trusts support midwife-led antenatal care varies, and there are differences in the role of the midwife in different places. At one end of the spectrum midwives act as clinical specialists; at the other, they support medical staff and chaperone women. Women's experience of antenatal clinics also varies from place to place. Some trusts run large hospital consultant clinics, with 50 or more women attending. Others offer a more personal service in community clinics, and where necessary, smaller hospital clinics targeted at clearly defined groups of women.

45. The differences between patterns of antenatal care are important because patterns determine the amount of choice and continuity of care available, and have cost implications. Many women prefer combinations of carers rather than single carers. In particular, the option of GP care is clearly important to some (Ref. 23). GPs are significant providers of services and yet decisions on the planning and delivery of services do not always take account of their contribution. Although many trusts offer alternative patterns of care, some do not or offer them only to highly restricted groups of women. Trusts should offer both options – antenatal care from obstetricians, GPs and midwives and antenatal care provided by, for example, midwives only – and should help women decide which is most appropriate for their needs and circumstances.

46. The different patterns of care are inevitably associated with different costs (Ref. 24). Traditional, obstetrician-led, shared care costs significantly more than GP/midwife care in the community. The staff costs of GP/midwife clinics are substantially lower than hospital consultant clinics, with a more than threefold variation between trusts visited, and much wider variations within the trusts themselves (Exhibit 8). There is often substantial variation in the numbers of women seen at the same clinic from week to week but staffing levels remain constant.

Exhibit 8
Costs of consultant and community antenatal clinic appointments

The staff costs of community clinics are substantially lower than those of consultant clinics.

*Community clinics include GP/ midwife and midwife only clinics.

Source: Audit Commission study sites (data unavailable at one trust)

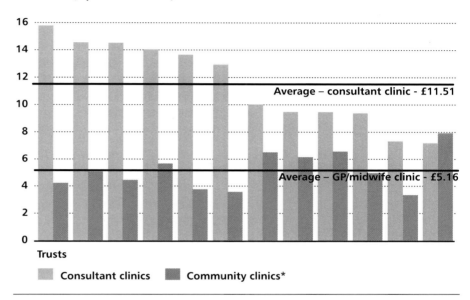

Staff costs (£ per woman seen)

Average – consultant clinic - £11.51

Average – GP/midwife clinic - £5.16

Trusts

■ **Consultant clinics**   ■ **Community clinics***

47. A recent randomised trial confirmed that routine specialist visits for women at low risk of complications are of little or no benefit and outcomes (for example, rates of antenatal diagnosis) are similar in hospital and community clinics (Ref. 25). Trusts should review the use of routine hospital attendances and encourage the option of community-based care for women with uncomplicated pregnancies, without compromising access to specialist opinions where and when they are needed (Case Study 1). Even for women

Case Study 1
Guidelines for identifying appropriate levels of service for antenatal care

Royal Berkshire and Battle Hospitals NHS Trust

At the Royal Berkshire and Battle NHS Trust, antenatal care has been GP/midwife-led since 1988. GPs and midwives carry out all antenatal checks unless there is a specific indication that the woman needs to see a consultant. Indications are listed in multi-professional guidelines, and include previous medical and obstetric history, and symptoms such as raised blood pressure.

All women visit the Royal Berkshire hospital or one of the local community hospitals for one scan, but they see the consultant only if they are under consultant care. Women also move from GP/midwife care to consultant care and back again if the problem is resolved.

'...women with complications in pregnancy may not be offered aspects of care... that are generally felt to be of value.'

for whom a medical opinion is sought, it should be possible (as with other specialties) to revert to management in a primary care setting (including midwifery care) once the specific problem has been resolved. Indeed, many trusts could substantially reduce the number of antenatal hospital attendances if they followed the example of those already offering a community-based approach. This would be more acceptable to many women, and would allow hospital clinics to provide a better service for those with complicated pregnancies.

48. A transfer of activity into community settings will not always be easy. Suitable locations may not exist. In these circumstances, some trusts have considered the alternative of more midwife-only clinics in the hospital, offering potential advantages of better continuity, smaller clinics and lower costs. In order to avoid risks of duplication and to make better use of clinical skills, they should review professional roles in antenatal clinics.

49. Trusts should also review the way that clinics operate and, although there has been great improvement in waiting times, many could do more to improve the running of antenatal clinics. Clinics should be organised as far as possible as 'one-stop shops' with all necessary services (such as blood testing and scanning) available at one visit. Sometimes this can be achieved simply by ensuring that hospital departments have co-ordinated opening hours and developing clear definitions of who does what. Lastly, trusts should ensure that they monitor the effect of any changes to the organisation of antenatal care on overall costs and on women's views.

Services for women with complications in pregnancy

50. Women whose pregnancies are complicated by medical conditions or obstetric problems have additional clinical needs, while their needs for social support are the same as or greater than those of other women. They therefore need better communication with professionals, more information and greater reassurance. Communication between professionals must also work well, and there is a need for good practical arrangements for co-ordinating the services.

51. Despite these needs, and the prominence that *Changing Childbirth* gave to them, women with complications in pregnancy may not be offered aspects of care such as continuity of carer and locally based services that are generally felt to be of value. Moreover, because these women are likely to be referred to a specialist centre, which may be some distance away, good communication is less rather than more likely. These factors may partly explain why they are less positive about maternity care than other women and express more dissatisfaction with the information provided.

52. A trust's capacity to provide specialist services for women with particular health problems will depend on the number of such women using its services. Different responses to their needs will be appropriate in different circumstances. It is not always possible to provide specialist services locally, but some trusts are attempting to tackle these issues (Box C).

Box C
Initiatives found in some trusts aimed at meeting the needs of women with complications or health problems in pregnancy

- ◆ a hospital-based midwifery team linked to a small medical team to provide continuity of medical and midwifery care;
- ◆ specialist midwives who retain contact with women and with their local carers to help women feel that support is ongoing;
- ◆ specialist antenatal clinics run jointly with physicians from other specialties. In smaller units the clinics occur less frequently;
- ◆ clinics co-ordinated with other specialties where a joint clinic is not possible; and
- ◆ peripheral consultant clinics away from the hospital setting, with fewer attendees and a less-pressured environment.

Number of antenatal checks

53.   The number of antenatal checks that a woman receives is based largely on a pattern of care originating in the 1920s (Ref. 26). There is little evidence that the number of checks is associated with the long-term health of mother or baby, but high levels of routine contact may have knock-on effects, with an increased likelihood of further antenatal assessment, ultrasound scans and hospital admission (Ref. 27). There are no current professional guidelines on appropriate levels of care, but the Government has recommended that provision of antenatal care be reviewed (Refs. 4, 5) and others have recommended fewer clinic visits for women at low risk of complications and have evaluated revised patterns of care (Refs. 27, 28) (Box D).

Box D
Traditional versus revised patterns of care for first-time mothers with uncomplicated pregnancies

Type of care	Up to 28 weeks gestation	28-36 weeks gestation	36+ weeks gestation
Traditional care (13 checks)	Monthly	Fortnightly	Weekly
Revised pattern of care (9 checks)	Booking at 12 weeks. Further checks at 16 weeks and 28 weeks	36 weeks	Weekly

Source: Adapted from Chamberlain, 1994 (Ref. 26)

54. Hospital policies suggest that women with uncomplicated pregnancies having their first baby should be offered between 7 and 13 antenatal checks. Many hospitals do not have a firm policy (Exhibit 9) and, in practice, patterns of care are usually based on traditional models of care (Box D). GPs, too, continue to offer a traditional pattern of care, with GPs surveyed by the Audit Commission typically recommending 12–13 antenatal checks (excluding scans).

55. The Commission estimates that providing the traditional pattern of antenatal checks recommended by current hospital policies rather than a reduced pattern, such as that suggested by the Welsh Office (Ref. 4), represents approximately £10 million of NHS resources.

56. However, reducing the number of antenatal checks will not be straightforward. As a first step, trusts must review the service currently being provided. This means that quality of data on the number of antenatal checks that women receive in practice must be improved. Trusts must define clinics' objectives and the timing and frequency of the activities needed to achieve them. In doing so, they should not forget the less tangible objectives of antenatal care, such as providing information, support and reassurance.

Exhibit 9
Recommended numbers of antenatal checks for women with uncomplicated pregnancies

Some trusts have moved away from traditional patterns of care.

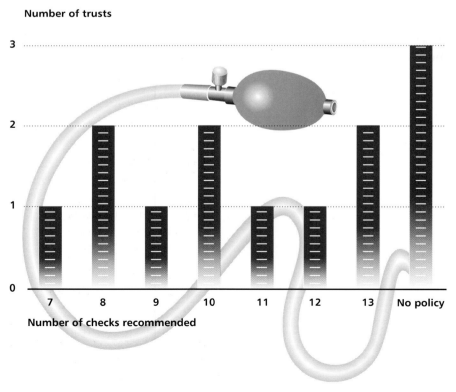

Number of trusts

Number of checks recommended

Note: Patterns of care are described for women having their first baby, up to and including 40 weeks gestation. Excludes appointments for scans or blood tests only.

Source: Audit Commission study sites

57. The persistence of high numbers of routine antenatal checks may be due to women's desire for contact with health professionals and anxiety about reduced contact (Ref. 27), a growing acceptance of the role of antenatal care in providing advice and reassurance and more care being provided in community settings, which women find more accessible. It may also be due to a lack of confidence or consensus among professionals. There may be a view that reducing the number of antenatal checks does not fit with providing woman-centred care, or that it may conflict with some other priority in the service. For example, attempts at improving 'continuity of carer' by providing care from only a limited number of midwives in a 'team' can mean that the planned number of antenatal contacts is high to ensure that women meet all of their carers.

58. Providing more care than is needed means poor use of resources which could be better targeted at improving information and support for women, particularly those with more complex needs. Efforts will be needed to identify effective forms of education and reassurance outside the traditional antenatal clinic. For example, some hospitals are establishing support groups for women; initially facilitated by a midwife, the intention is that these groups will eventually be run by women themselves. Others have midwives who take an increasing role in educating women about appropriate use of services while maintaining high levels of satisfaction among those women who are using the service.

Clinical content of antenatal checks

59. If the number of antenatal visits is to be reduced, it is essential that the checks that take place provide effective clinical care. This will require careful definition and organisation, and the implementation of policies should be monitored. Routine clinical activity in antenatal checks include tests to assess the progress of the pregnancy and detect problems in the health of the mother or baby, and screening for fetal abnormalities.

Routine tests

60. A wide range of tests is currently carried out in antenatal clinics. These vary from procedures such as weighing all pregnant women, which are of limited clinical value when repeated routinely, through to essential tests such as monitoring urine protein levels and blood pressure measurements to screen for pre-eclampsia.

61. The extent to which different procedures are currently carried out varies considerably. Some of the hospitals visited by the Audit Commission have stopped routine weighing of pregnant women while others still weigh all women at every clinic attendance. But there is also variation in the levels of essential screening tests. Records show that in some trusts only two-thirds of women attending are having their urine and blood pressure checked. There is also wide variation in practice between clinics in the same trust.

'...purchasers should take the lead in policy-making, specifying in contracts the screening programme to be purchased...'

62. Of course the failure to record tests does not necessarily mean that they are not happening. It is possible, for example, that in some of these cases women are checking their own urine and, for this or other reasons, test results are not being recorded. And if some antenatal attendances are specifically to provide support, information and reassurance, this may also explain low rates of testing. But whatever the explanation, it is important that trusts decide which tests are essential and then set up careful monitoring mechanisms to ensure that they are being applied.

Screening for fetal abnormality

63. A range of different kinds of screening tests can be used to detect the risk of fetal abnormality early in pregnancy. These include various blood tests (for example, serum screening for Down's syndrome) as well as ultrasound scanning. There is a lack of professional consensus on the value of routine scanning in early pregnancy (as opposed to scans that are triggered by specific clinical indications)(Ref. 29), and there is substantial variation in normal practice across western Europe. In the UK it has become a routine part of care for all women (Ref. 30) (99 per cent of women in the Audit Commission survey having had an ultrasound scan).

64. Use of these technologies is growing rapidly, due to both greater supply and demand. Clinicians frequently establish screening tests and women are also increasingly demanding these technologies of their own volition. This demand is sometimes fuelled by a positive view of the benefits (which include reassurance and providing valuable information about their babies) and because the practical problems or drawbacks associated with screening tests are not widely understood.

65. Many of these tests carry a range of potential problems for women and their families, including psychological and emotional ones (Refs. 31, 32). Like any screening tests, they miss some cases and raise some false alarms, sometimes giving uncertain results that require further tests. They therefore have the potential to cause great anxiety. Add to that their costs, and it is perhaps not surprising that many trusts are not providing all of these screening tests or are providing them only to restricted groups. Some trusts do not have a clear policy and leave it up to individual clinicians to make decisions about screening. In others, women are being given inadequate information about the purpose and possible meaning of tests, and are taking decisions about whether to have them without being fully informed.

66. As a first step, purchasers should take the lead in policy-making, specifying in contracts the screening programme to be purchased, following discussion with clinicians. There should be clear and explicit policies on such tests, including the availability of testing, provision of information and support to families, and arrangements for monitoring and multi-professional audit. They need to base their decisions on factors such as the age and ethnic profile of the population, the wishes and views of local service users, the opinions of clinicians, and resource constraints. A few trusts have tackled some of these issues; for example, by altering the programme of screening on offer in response to the systematic audit of its success. However, given the difficulties that trusts and purchasers are experiencing and the rapidly changing nature of screening technology, this may be an area where national guidance would be beneficial.

67. It is essential that policy on screening and scanning dovetails with other policies for antenatal care, to ensure that the knock-on effects on other parts of the service are properly considered. For example, do new screening tests require antenatal contact at a specific gestation that is not in line with current policy? Will screening provision mean that an extra hospital contact is needed because of lack of local expertise in information provision? Are there good practical links between disciplines in relation to screening?

68. It is likely that improving access to accurate information about screening tests will help to reduce their drawbacks. Initiatives aimed at producing user-friendly, well researched information for both women and professionals (such as those published by Midwives Information and Resource Services (MIDIRS) (Ref. 33)) are welcome. Purchasers and providers have a responsibility to evaluate the arrangements for information provision, since the best way of doing this is currently unclear. Responsibilities for provision of information, and for evaluation and audit of screening, need to be clarified. *Changing Childbirth* emphasised the need for a review of arrangements for counselling in relation to screening tests, and a review in this area is currently being undertaken by the Royal College of Obstetricians and Gynaecologists Audit Unit (Ref. 34).

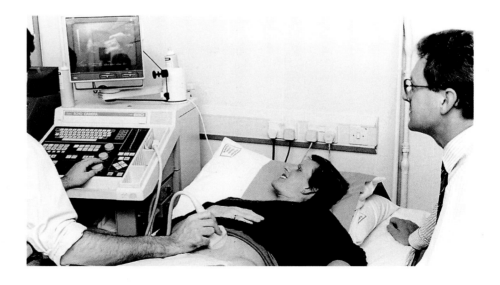

Recommendations

Clinicians and managers in trusts should:

1 pay attention to the special needs of women with complicated pregnancies for good communication and support.

2 develop antenatal policies that are flexible but that aim to make best use of the available resources for the whole population of users of maternity services.

3 agree guidelines for antenatal assessment and protocols for referral with their local GPs.

4 review the number of checks that they routinely offer to women at low risk of complications in pregnancy; adjust it, if necessary, to the recommended safe levels; and monitor the actual number of times that women are seen in practice.

5 review routine attendance at consultant clinics in hospital and aim to provide as much antenatal care as possible in the community.

6 make sure that women always have access to specialist services when they need it, and that once they have received a specialist opinion, their care reverts back to the community once the specific issue has been resolved.

7 target specialist obstetric care, which costs more than midwife-led and GP/midwife care, at the women who most need it.

8 avoid duplication of doctors' and midwives' skills in clinics and develop guidelines for who does what.

9 review clinical procedures in antenatal clinics, and make sure that all care given is known to be effective.

10 agree standards for information giving and counselling for antenatal screening, and monitor their implementation.

Commissioners should:

11   work closely with GPs and trusts to improve the oral and written information provided to pregnant women about all aspects of their care, including who will provide it, where it will take place and what it will involve.

12   take the lead in determining the kinds of screening and scanning that will be available to the population.

The NHS Executive should:

13   prioritise research into effective and efficient ways of meeting women's needs for information about services, and antenatal advice and support.

14   support commissioners by developing a national framework for local policies on antenatal screening and scanning.

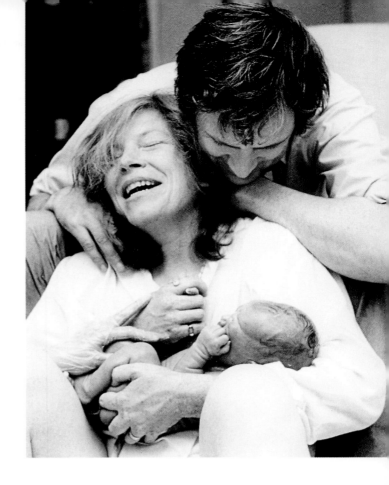

3 Care of Women in Labour and Birth

Trusts face a number of challenges in providing care for women in labour. They must ensure that clinical practice is based on the best available evidence, and that levels of medical intervention are appropriate.

As far as possible, trusts should also aim for childbirth to be a satisfying experience: emotional and social support contribute to this and can reduce the need for medical intervention. However, some women don't feel informed and involved in key decisions. Others describe a lack of professional support when in labour, or describe seeing a large numbers of different professional staff.

The wide variation in rates of medical intervention are a cause for concern. Avoiding unnecessary interventions is important. Women who have operative deliveries are less satisfied with their care, feel less well supported and suffer increased postnatal ill-health. High levels of intervention introduce additional costs to the NHS. Careful monitoring and good ongoing review are needed to ensure that care is provided in the most effective way.

Introduction

69. Trusts face a number of challenges in providing care for women in labour and birth. Of primary importance is the safety of mothers and babies. This means ensuring that clinical practice is based on the best available evidence, and that levels of medical intervention are appropriate. However, safety is not the only factor. It is also widely recognised that professional staff have a duty to ensure that, as far as possible, childbirth is a satisfying experience for mothers as well as a safe event for both mothers and babies. There is evidence that emotional and social support contribute to making childbirth a satisfying experience and can also reduce the need for medical intervention (Ref. 35). Providing clinically effective services as well as meeting women's wishes and needs are important objectives that run alongside the need to make best use of resources.

70. There is a range of options available for the care of women in labour regardless of the pattern of antenatal care provided: women can deliver in a hospital consultant unit (currently 97 per cent of the total); a GP or midwife-led unit (around 1 per cent in the Audit Commission survey); or at home (around 2 per cent). Hospital labour wards usually consist of a number of single delivery rooms (between five and 22 at the hospitals visited), one or two dedicated obstetric theatres and, sometimes, additional beds for the initial assessment or care of women in early labour. In addition, some trusts have birthing pool suites and others have 'home from home' rooms (either on the labour ward or elsewhere), which offer the option of a more domestic environment for labour and delivery. Different combinations of professionals are likely to be involved according to the place of birth, the complexity of the delivery and, sometimes, women's preferences.

71. Although, nationally, around 2 per cent of births take place at home, this varies widely around the country. In the trusts visited during this study, the proportion of births taking place at home ranged from less than 0.5 per cent to over 4 per cent. Although small in number, home births receive a great deal of attention, sometimes taking on symbolic importance as an indicator of the extent of flexibility in the maternity services. In the vast majority of cases, midwives employed by trusts care for women having babies at home (82 per cent of GPs in the Audit Commission survey had had no involvement with home births in the previous year). For trusts where demand for home births is growing, midwives' lack of familiarity with home deliveries can present particular challenges for the organisation and training of staff.

'Providing clinically effective services as well as meeting women's wishes and needs are important objectives that run alongside the need to make best use of resources.'

72. Most women take a decision early in pregnancy on where to give birth. It is an important decision, because each trust has its own policies and practices. More than 80 per cent of women surveyed said that they already knew where they wanted their babies to be born at the start of their antenatal care. It is difficult to tell how much awareness women have of the options that are available. Certainly some options, such as GP units, are available to relatively few women (Exhibit 10). However, 17 per cent of women in this study reported that they had had the option of a home birth, an option which has in the past been thought to be greatly limited. Prospective parents need good information on the range of options available.

73. This chapter reviews some of the key areas of care of women in labour and childbirth. It begins with factors that will affect all women: the need for privacy and comfort, and for pain relief appropriate to individual needs. It goes on to review the efficiency and effectiveness with which midwives are deployed. Lastly, it considers medical interventions, which are of concern to many professionals, affect outcomes and have an impact on women's satisfaction with their care, as well as having major resource implications.

Exhibit 10
Women's perceptions of the options available for place of delivery

Some options are not thought to be widely available.

Note: Numbers do not total 100 per cent as respondents could select more than one option.
*Domino = 'Domiciliary In and Out' – a system in which community midwives visit women in labour at home, escort them into hospital for delivery, and transfer them home following a short (less than 24-hour) hospital stay.

Source: Audit Commission survey of recent mothers (N = 2,375)

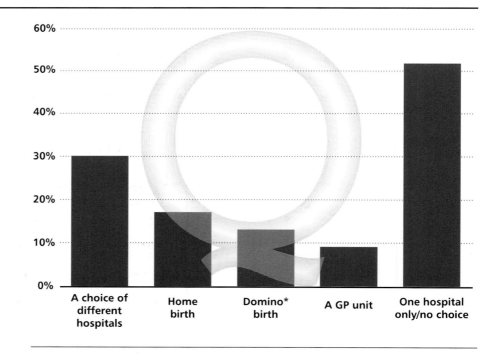

Caring for women in labour

74. Focusing maternity services on women's individual requirements as well as on achieving safe delivery means that professionals need to involve them fully in decisions about their care, both in pregnancy and in labour. Women's responses to the Audit Commission survey indicate variable progress in this area. Around 40 per cent report having had a say in decisions to induce or accelerate labour, but only half this number felt that they were fully involved in decisions about how the baby was monitored or whether to have an episiotomy (Exhibit 11).

75. Many pregnant women and their partners know in advance, from childbirth preparation classes and other sources, what sort of birth they would ideally like to have. More than half the women surveyed knew whether they did or did not want particular medical procedures. In many cases, these preferences had been written into a birth plan or their casenotes. When women's preferences are not met, they are less likely to say that they were treated with kindness, understanding and respect. Although failure to meet preferences is usually because of changes in medical circumstances, it occasionally occurs simply as an oversight.

Exhibit 11
Involvement of women in decisions during labour

Some women do not feel involved in key decisions during labour.

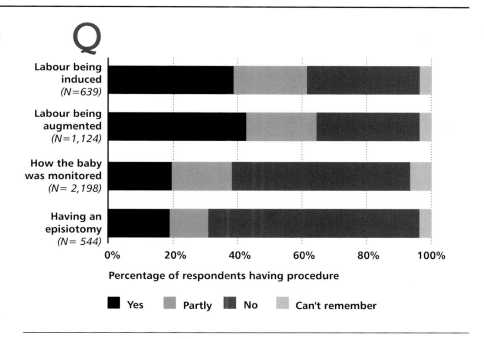

Source: Audit Commission survey of recent mothers

'All recipients of healthcare should be treated in a way which meets their clinical needs without compromising dignity and privacy. But, in the day-to-day running of busy labour wards, these needs can be overlooked.'

76. All recipients of healthcare should be treated in a way which meets their clinical needs without compromising dignity and privacy. But, in the day-to-day running of busy labour wards, these needs can be overlooked. Examples at one trust visited included labour rooms where the doors were propped open, leaving only a curtain for privacy, and women in labour were being asked personal questions in public areas on the labour ward. At another trust, women are moved when they are in established labour if an epidural is required, and companions are routinely excluded while epidurals are put in place. Trusts also vary in their flexibility with regard to eating and drinking in labour, bathing in labour, and the presence of birth companions.

Pain relief

77. Many women need help in coping with pain in labour but for some it is important to manage without pharmacological pain relief. The most frequently used combination of methods of pain relief is inhaled analgesia (such as entonox) along with intra-muscular analgesia (such as pethidine), although there is great variation in methods of pain relief used from trust to trust. Different methods have both benefits and disadvantages and many women have strong preferences.

78. Around one-quarter of the women surveyed had epidural analgesia, either alone or together with other methods of pain relief. The availability of epidural analgesia varies. For example, interviews with professionals at one trust visited suggested that up to one-quarter of women who requested epidural analgesia in labour did not get it, despite a '24-hour epidural service'.

79. It is important that women are given good information antenatally about the pros and cons of different sorts of pain relief, as well as a realistic assessment of their chances of having access to their method of choice. To do this, trusts will need to monitor the use of different forms of pain relief, and waiting times, particularly for epidurals. It is also important that the easy availability of pharmacological methods of pain relief does not reduce the emphasis on the role of emotional support for women.

Facilities

80. Hospitals vary in the standards of basic facilities for women in labour. And in some there are major differences between the best and the worst facilities on offer. Some of the trusts visited provide birthing pools, others encourage women to hire them, others accept rather than encourage it, and some do not allow it at all. While some women may be offered luxurious birthing pool suites, others in the same hospital may have to compete with four or more other women for access to a bath or shower on the delivery suite, or can spend substantial time in labour in multi-bedded bays alongside other women.

81. There are also equity considerations. Local policies in some trusts specify that women labouring in birthing pools must be attended by two midwives throughout their labour. This can have implications for the level of professional support available to other women on the labour ward, especially if the birthing pool is some distance from the main labour ward.

82. Within any trust, the physical properties of the facilities themselves and the attitudes of staff will influence women in labour. The arrangement of furniture and equipment in labour wards communicates a message to women about what is seen as 'the norm'. Although midwives at trusts visited assured us that they were happy to support women's preferences for managing their labours as they wished, the fixed lay-out of all the rooms and lack of visible alternatives might make it difficult for women to ask for changes to be made.

83. Labour ward staff could help by experimenting with different ways of setting out delivery rooms, and by making alternative equipment more easily accessible. This is an area that could be emphasised in tours of labour wards for expectant parents and in written information.

Midwife staffing

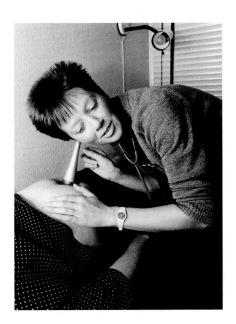

84. Staff are the major resource in providing care for women in labour: midwifery is the largest part of this resource, accounting for 86 per cent of basic staff costs at trusts visited. Most women need continuous professional support throughout labour (Ref. 36), and for the most part, this is likely to be provided by a midwife. The extent to which women are left without support during labour is of concern, with around one-quarter of women surveyed describing being worried when left without professional support during labour.

85. Trusts need to ensure that staffing levels are appropriate so that there are sufficient staff to provide a safe service and adequate support to women. In labour and birth, when women's needs for support can be acute, good quality personal support has been shown to have a significant impact in enhancing maternal well-being and satisfaction (Ref. 36).

Organisation of staff

86. Problems in staffing labour wards are common. Only three of the 13 trusts visited have reviewed their midwifery staffing on the labour ward in relation to indicators of need or workload, and a further two were running team midwifery across the service as a whole which meant that staffing numbers on the labour ward more closely reflected the number of women cared for. Although, on paper, all but five of the trusts have sufficient staff on the labour ward to provide one-to-one support from qualified midwives, this level of support was in practice not being achieved most of the time (Exhibit 12). This failure to provide the right level of support is due mainly to fluctuations in workload, but is exacerbated by inflexible deployment of staff, failing to relate to peaks and troughs in activity.

87. Trusts can take several steps to improve the flexibility of labour ward staffing. They should review the levels of midwifery staffing overall and the provision of support staff, and how staff are deployed in response to workload, taking into account the case-mix as well as peaks and troughs in activity. Some trusts rotate staff from community settings on to the labour ward. Although such rotation is usually intended to help staff to maintain their skills in caring for women in labour it could also, potentially, help to provide extra flexibility in staffing.

Exhibit 12
Proportion of occasions when one-to-one midwifery support was possible on labour wards

One-to-one midwifery support was not being achieved most of the time.

*Proportion of occasions when 1.15:1 staffing levels achieved – eight-hourly intervals over a two-week period (1.15:1 is used to allow one-to-one support, plus 15 per cent for management and other duties).

Source: Audit Commission study sites (data unavailable at one trust)

Percentage of time points over a two-week period*

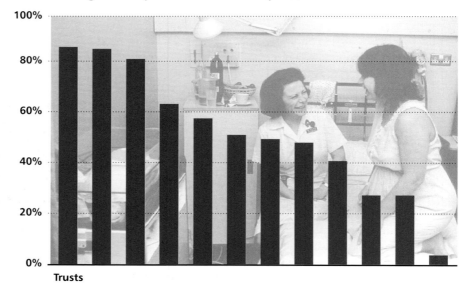

Trusts

88. One trust had a more flexible method of matching staff to actual workload (Exhibit 13), achieving desired staffing levels on over 80 per cent of occasions. This trust had organised all midwives (apart from a very small core staff) into teams. One of the objectives of team and caseload midwifery is to ensure that staff are available to women when they are needed. If successful, this can prove an extremely useful way of ensuring that labour wards are appropriately staffed without detracting from the quality of care elsewhere. However, not all caseload schemes achieve this flexibility, partly because they frequently provide care for only a small proportion of the women receiving care, running alongside traditional shift-based systems of organising staff.

89. Some trusts also draw in staff from antenatal and postnatal wards when labour wards are busy. While some flexibility of staffing is desirable, it is important that the demands of one area do not compromise the quality of care in another.

Exhibit 13
Matching staffing to workload

Some trusts are more successful than others in matching staffing to workload.

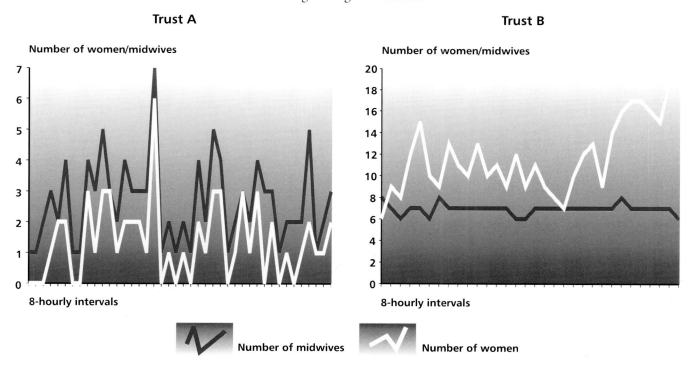

Note: Staffing and activity (number of women) at eight-hourly intervals over a two-week period.
Source: Audit Commission study sites

Continuity of carer

90. Some women express a desire for continuity of carer in labour, either from a midwife they have met before or simply from the same midwife throughout labour (Chapter 1). Yet women are often looked after by a large number of different professionals during labour. Although this is in part due to the complexity of some labours and deliveries, it can also be due to the way staffing is organised, to hospital routines, or to a failure to acknowledge the need for continuity. Clearly it can be difficult to achieve continuity in long labours. But for labour lasting less than, say, 12 hours, it ought to be possible to arrange continuity from two or, at most, three midwives. Despite this, more than one-quarter of women at trusts in the study who spent less than 12 hours on the labour ward were cared for by four or more different midwives. There was also substantial variation between trusts in their success at achieving continuity (Exhibit 14).

91. Sometimes the involvement of students can affect continuity of carer. Staff have to be trained, but there has to be a careful balancing of their need for education and training and women's needs for a private and supportive environment. Methods of training medical and midwifery staff should be designed to minimise disruption for women: for example, case discussions between medical and midwifery staff involved in the care of individual women can be used instead of ward rounds, in which all labouring women are seen routinely by groups of unfamiliar professionals. And, of course, where students are involved, women's permission must be obtained at all times.

Exhibit 14
Continuity of carer in labour – labours lasting 12 hours or less

There was substantial variation between trusts in providing continuity of carer in labour.

Note: Staffing records of 200 births at each trust (analysis of labours in women who spent 12 hours or less on the labour ward)

Source: Audit Commission study sites (data unavailable at one trust)

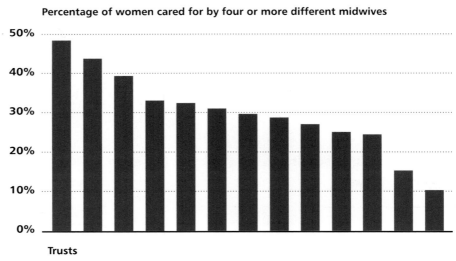

Percentage of women cared for by four or more different midwives

Trusts

Medical interventions – providing effective care

92. Over time, doctors and midwives have developed knowledge and skills in when and how to intervene in the process of labour to improve its outcome. Examples include techniques to induce labour when babies need to be born urgently; for example, for some women suffering from pre-eclampsia. Operative methods of delivery such as caesarean section, forceps and ventouse (vacuum extractor) have also been an important development in obstetrics, saving the lives of many women and their babies. Of women surveyed by the Audit Commission, 17 per cent had a delivery by caesarean section, 6 per cent had a forceps delivery and 5 per cent a ventouse delivery.

93. Most such procedures carry benefits, risks and costs. While in some situations, the indications for certain medical interventions are very clear, in others they are less clear cut. There are inter-relationships between some interventions – for example, the use of routine continuous electronic fetal monitoring increases the likelihood of subsequent operative delivery independently of other factors (Exhibit 15). The appropriateness of medical intervention in each case should, therefore, be a carefully considered joint decision by the professional staff and the woman concerned. In addition, some women will themselves have strong preferences regarding (wanting or not wanting) particular procedures in labour.

Exhibit 15
Inter-relationships between medical interventions in labour

Some interventions increase the likelihood of others.

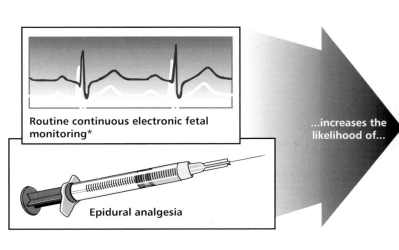
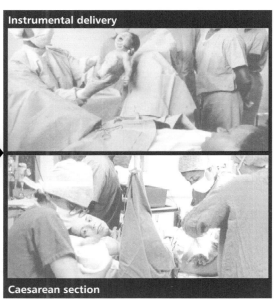

*Routine continuous electronic fetal monitoring without fetal blood sampling
Source: Audit Commission (Refs. 37, 38)

94. There are wide variations in intervention rates both nationally and internationally, even between countries of similar levels of economic development, and for some specific medical indications (for example, caesarean section for breech presentation, or for previous caesarean section (Ref. 39)). For other medical indications, research is hampered by the lack of consistency in definitions of conditions such as 'failure to progress' or 'fetal distress' and by differing thresholds for using these diagnoses. Differences in levels of intervention are influenced by the nature of the population served (case-mix) but also by a range of other factors.

95. Most recently, the Clinical Standards Advisory Group (CSAG) identified widely varying practices in the care of a selected group of women without pre-existing risk factors. The high levels of some procedures suggest that they are being carried out on a routine basis (Ref. 40) and that it is local policies rather than professional judgement that explain the frequency of some interventions. Examples include vaginal examinations and artificial rupture of membranes. The CSAG review recommended that multi-disciplinary policies on the management of normal labour were needed to clarify practice.

96. Avoiding unnecessary interventions is important for a variety of reasons. Women having instrumental deliveries, for example, describe reduced levels of satisfaction and confidence, feel less well supported and suffer increased postnatal ill health.

97. High levels of medical intervention are also of concern because of their cost to the NHS. Women who have operative deliveries stay longer in hospital and need more care. Estimates by Clark (1991) suggest that a caesarean section costs £760 more than a vaginal delivery (Ref. 41), so every 1 per cent increase in the rate of caesarean section costs the NHS over £5 million per annum.

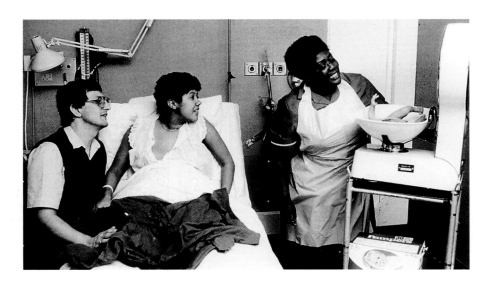

Instrumental deliveries

98. There are wide variations both nationally and internationally in rates of assisted vaginal delivery (Ref. 42). Current professional guidance suggests that, in general, where an assisted vaginal delivery is required, ventouse should be used in preference to forceps as the instrument of first choice (Ref. 43) although other factors, such as the training of the operator, need to be taken into account in the short term. Women whose babies are delivered by ventouse generally suffer less pain and injury to the genital tract than those delivered using forceps (Ref. 44). There is little evidence as yet to distinguish between forceps and ventouse in the long-term outcomes for babies and ongoing audit will be needed. Trusts vary in the extent to which ventouse is the preferred option (Exhibit 16) although most are making progress in this direction.

Caesarean sections

99. The use of caesarean section has increased in most developed countries to a level that concerns clinicians (Refs. 45, 46). Caesarean section carries major benefits for some women and babies, but also risks – for example, of operative injury and complications of anaesthesia. Post-operative recovery can also be lengthy. Concerns among professionals about risk of litigation are likely to have fuelled the increase in the use of caesarean section. But although there is general consensus that levels of caesarean section are higher than are clinically required, there is currently no consensus about

Exhibit 16
Instrumental delivery rates at study sites

Trusts vary in the extent to which ventouse is the preferred option in instrumental delivery.

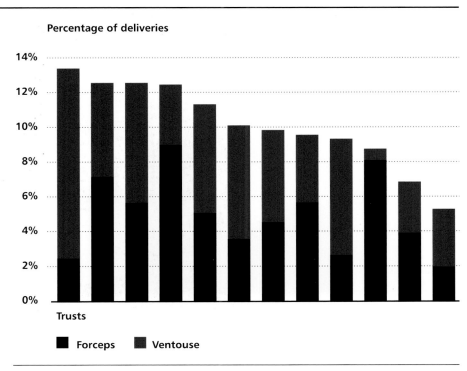

Source: Audit Commission study sites (data unavailable at one trust)

the optimum. Caesarean sections at trusts visited in the study ranged from 11 per cent to 18 per cent of deliveries (Exhibit 17) and vary more than twofold nationally. The extent to which differences are due to case-mix, as opposed to other factors, is unknown.

100. Both medical and non-medical factors, including professional norms and fear of litigation, are major influences on rates of caesarean section (Ref. 39). This is also an area where there is sometimes said to be a conflict between women's choice and the most effective and efficient form of care. Obstetricians report that women are occasionally choosing this as their preferred form of delivery, their wishes influencing the decision to perform caesarean section (Ref. 47). This could potentially place an upward pressure on overall rates. Some are hopeful that good information and discussion with women, coupled with the general drive of the consumer movement to reduce interventions, will contain the rates. The likely overall impact of each of these factors is unclear, and most trusts do not have a clear response to women requesting this procedure.

Exhibit 17
Caesarean section rates

The use of caesarean section at trusts visited ranged from 11 per cent to 18 per cent of deliveries.

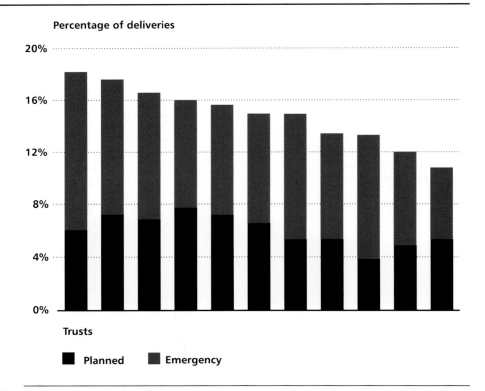

Percentage of deliveries

Trusts

■ **Planned**   ■ **Emergency**

*Source: Audit Commission study sites
(data unavailable at two trusts)*

Episiotomies, tears and stitches

101. In recent years, with a general acceptance that over-use of episiotomy should be discouraged, episiotomy rates have declined. Twenty-seven per cent of women surveyed had had an episiotomy (19 per cent of those having a spontaneous vaginal delivery), but two-thirds felt that they had not had any say in the decision. Although this is a procedure which is likely to take place at a time when discussion and explanation are difficult, it is likely that improved emphasis on information provision, and the opportunity to discuss birth events postnatally, are likely to improve women's feelings of involvement. There are substantial variations in episiotomy rates between trusts (Exhibit 18), and even between professionals within trusts (Ref. 48).

Improving the use of medical interventions

102. Action should be taken to help women who need medical interventions and operative deliveries. Reduced maternal satisfaction should not be accepted as inevitable, and obstetricians, midwives and childbirth educators should try to identify possible ways of preventing disappointment and feelings of failure in these women. Good information and the opportunity to discuss birth events in detail with a professional who is familiar with the individual circumstances are important.

Exhibit 18
Episiotomy rates at study sites

Episiotomy rates have declined, but substantial variations remain in the rates at different trusts.

Source: Audit Commission study sites (data unavailable at four trusts visited)

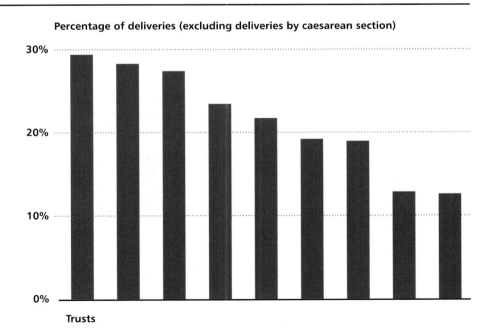

Percentage of deliveries (excluding deliveries by caesarean section)

Trusts

'While medical factors are a major influence on levels of intervention, non-medical factors... play at least as great, if not a greater part.'

103. What can be done to ensure that all interventions are appropriate, and to reduce rates where they are not? As a first step, it is essential that good quality national data are available. The Hospital Episode System (HES) has been severely criticised for being both incomplete and inaccurate (Ref. 49) and should be targeted for improvement. Other data, such as those routinely collected by the Royal College of Obstetricians and Gynaecologists (RCOG) are a valuable source of information, and should be more widely available as a tool for audit, published annually on a trust-by-trust basis (Ref. 50).

104. Methods of adjusting data to reflect local case-mix, such as the 'standard primipara' (a subgroup of women fulfilling certain criteria, who would be expected to have similar rates of intervention) should be used to improve the robustness of comparison of clinical practice from trust to trust (Ref. 51).

105. The next step is to understand and tackle the factors that cause unduly high intervention rates. While medical factors are a major influence on levels of intervention, non-medical factors (such as fear of litigation, professional norms and convenience) play at least as great, if not a greater part (Ref. 39). Women's choices may also have an effect and they need clear and unbiased information on the pros and cons of various interventions. Trusts should ensure that the impact of maternal requests for procedures is well documented, and develop policies to support clinical staff in this sensitive area.

106. It is important to identify obstacles to change. These can include the skills and confidence of individual clinicians, and concern whether an intervention is needed as well as which is the most appropriate intervention to undertake. A particular problem can arise when a new procedure is introduced which senior staff do not feel confident to carry out themselves or to train and educate junior staff in its use. Managers must recognise training and education needs when changes in practice are advisable. Recent success in increasing the use of the ventouse shows that progress can be made.

107. Ongoing audit and peer review can assist with the change process (Refs. 52, 53). This continuous assessment process should be interdisciplinary, and be given a high priority by purchasers and trusts. Attempts should be made to reach a consensus about standards for audit, and clinical guidelines should be developed out of the audit process (Case Study 2). Efforts to tackle rates of caesarean section have often focused on improving knowledge of research findings. While this is necessary, other measures may also be needed (Ref. 45). Enthusiastic individuals who act as 'educational leaders' may be one way forward. Detailed retrospective review by obstetricians at all levels to judge the necessity of every caesarean section has also been suggested (Ref. 54) and is an approach being used at some of the trusts visited.

Case Study 2
Multidisciplinary clinical audit of care in labour and delivery

North Staffordshire Hospital NHS Trust

The North Staffordshire Hospital NHS Trust launched a project in July 1995 with the aim of producing 20 evidence-based guidelines for use in pregnancy and childbirth. Topics for the guidelines were chosen following a multi-disciplinary meeting of clinicians and service users. Funding for the project was obtained from the Region through a joint bid by the trust and the health authority.

Nine of the guidelines relate to care of women in labour and delivery. Of these, five promote safer care for women and babies, one looks at better continuity through a reduction in the number of carers, and the remaining three aim to prevent unnecessary or more damaging interventions.

Individuals or groups of staff – including obstetricians and midwives – take responsibility for a particular guideline: collecting baseline data on the standard, preparing the guideline itself, training staff and re-auditing at specified time intervals. They share the results with their midwifery and obstetric colleagues at monthly audit meetings, and with the health authority every quarter.

The trust has managed to move towards its targets in the first 15 months. Some examples are shown below.

Audit standard	Baseline audit finding	Current audit findings (October 1996)
100% of women with an uncomplicated breech presentation at term should be offered external cephalic version	50%	84%
95% of assisted vaginal deliveries should be with the ventouse rather than the forceps	80%	83%
100% of women with massive obstetric haemorrhage should be managed according to the relevant local guidelines	25%	77%
100% of women having caesarean section should receive prophylactic antibiotics	75%	91%
100% of women with severe pre-eclampsia, HELLP or eclampsia should be managed according to the relevant local guidelines	30%	53%
100% of mothers delivering at 26-34 weeks should have received two doses of steroids up to seven days before delivery	40%	85%

Recommendations

Clinicians and managers in trusts should:

1 do more to help women feel involved in decisions about their care. They should make sure that women have all the necessary information and that they understand what is happening to them.

2 help women and their partners prepare for labour by providing information in advance that will help them assess their options for pain relief.

3 use tours of the labour ward and written information to emphasise the extent to which women should feel they have a say over all aspects of their care.

4 ensure that arrangements for providing training and education to doctors and midwives are compatible with protecting women's privacy and dignity.

5 ensure that women are not left without professional support in labour when they need or want it.

6 aim to provide one-to-one midwifery support for women in established labour.

7 review levels of staffing and introduce more flexible methods of staff deployment to allow better matching of fluctuating demand on the labour ward.

8 aim to reduce the number of different staff involved in the care of individual women to a minimum. For labours lasting 12 hours or less, no more than two or three different midwives should normally be involved.

9 make sure that midwives organise their work to maximise continuity of carer in labour for individual women.

10 ensure that the impact of maternal requests for procedures (such as caesarean section) is well-documented.

11   collect data on selected groups of women, such as the standard primipara, that will allow them to compare their own intervention rates with those of trusts caring for similar populations.

12   make sure that women receive accurate, unbiased and complete information about the risks and benefits of interventions.

13   ensure that clinicians have access to training and education and keep up to date.

14   establish multidisciplinary clinical audit and peer review.

Commissioners with trusts should:

15   make sure that they provide women with information on all the options for where to give birth.

16   keep rates of medical interventions in labour under review while monitoring changes in case-mix.

The NHS Executive should:

17   improve the quality of nationally collected maternity information on the Hospital Episode System and ensure that the data are disseminated.

18   devise, together with the RCOG, systematic and standard means of collecting case-mix data, and should encourage trusts to use them.

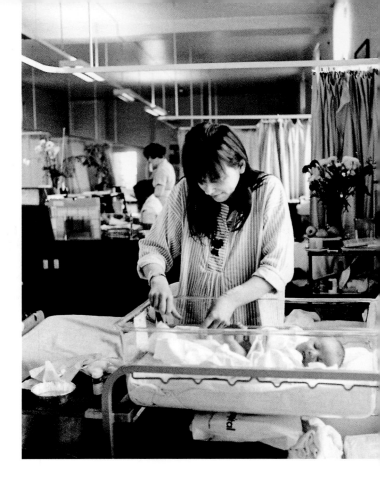

4 Care of Women after Childbirth and the Care of Newborn Babies

Women make more negative comments about hospital postnatal services than any other aspects of their maternity care. Resources allocated to postnatal care vary substantially; trusts should review the efficiency and quality of postnatal hospital care and target postnatal community services where they are most needed.

Trusts should have flexible policies on hospital stays and consult women about what happens to them. Women frequently report lack of support and conflicting advice on infant feeding; trusts should establish a breastfeeding policy and collect information on breastfeeding rates.

Some sick babies are looked after in neonatal units. These differ substantially in levels of activity and staffing, with activity at some trusts failing to match levels recommended to maintain clinical skills. Purchasers and trusts need to plan together the extent to which neonatal services will be concentrated in larger regional units as opposed to smaller local units.

Some neonatal units could also do more to support parents, recognising their vital role in the care of their babies by welcoming and involving them.

Introduction

108. Following birth, women need time to recover physically and emotionally, to establish feeding and, with their partners, to develop relationships with their babies. They need to be confident that any problems with the baby will be detected, and that appropriate care and treatment are available. For some babies this might mean special care on the ward; for others, care in a specialist facility or neonatal unit (NNU). In such cases, or where a baby dies, parents and relatives need sympathetic care, good information and ongoing support.

109. But recovery and adjustment to parenthood are often hampered by the mothers' own health problems (Exhibit 19). More than 85 per cent of women have reported at least one health problem postnatally in hospital and more than three-quarters of women are still reporting problems more than eight weeks after delivery (Ref. 55). Some women experience problems many years after childbirth. Postnatal health problems are closely associated with particular interventions during delivery (Refs. 56, 57). For all these reasons, care during the postnatal period must be properly planned and delivered.

Exhibit 19
Postnatal health problems

Many women report health problems following childbirth.

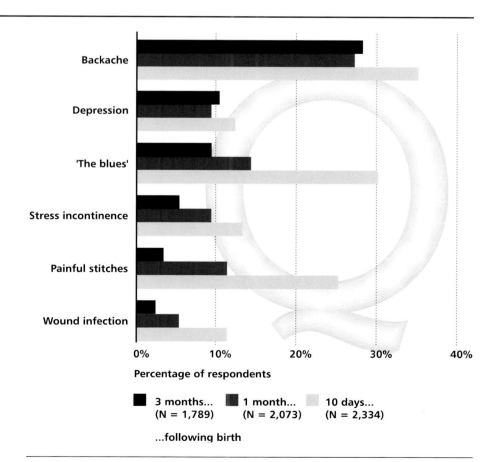

Percentage of respondents

■ 3 months... (N = 1,789)	■ 1 month... (N = 2,073)	□ 10 days... (N = 2,334)

...following birth

Source: Audit Commission survey of recent mothers

110. Most women having babies in hospital will receive some postnatal care on a hospital ward. Following discharge from hospital, midwives have a legal responsibility to care for mothers and babies for at least ten, and up to 28 days after birth. In practice, this means a variable number of home visits by midwives. These visits are usually daily for the first few days. Many women are also visited at home by their GPs. Health visitors usually take women and babies on to their caseload around the 10th day. This report does not examine the activities of health visitors.

111. Most new mothers have a six-week postnatal check, usually carried out by GPs, which has a largely physical emphasis, although it is also said to be for providing reassurance, an opportunity to discuss delivery events, advice on contraception and breastfeeding and for responding to concerns about the baby (Refs 58, 59). There is little evidence on the extent to which such needs are being addressed by these checks, and more research is needed.

112. There is in any case some uncertainty about what postnatal care is aiming to achieve – whether it is solely to prevent and treat immediate health problems in mother and baby or whether it is aiming to enhance the overall experience, giving mothers time to recover and get to know their babies, possibly avoiding other problems later. Perhaps because of this uncertainty, there is considerable variation in the nature of postnatal care and the levels of resources. Women make more negative comments about hospital postnatal services than any other aspects of their care (Appendix 1, Table 10).

113. This chapter looks first at the efficient use of postnatal resources – length of stay and staffing levels in hospital, and home visiting by midwives. It then considers some aspects of quality – hospital facilities and services to help with infant feeding. Lastly, following on from earlier work by the Audit Commission (Ref. 60) it looks at a range of issues involved in the care of sick babies in neonatal units (NNUs).

Efficient postnatal care

Length of hospital stay

114. The time that women stay in hospital after giving birth has been decreasing for many years. However, there is still considerable variation between localities and trusts. Part of the variation reflects different levels of intervention. Caesarean section, for example, nearly trebles the average length of stay (with an average length of stay of almost seven days compared to 2.5 days for normal deliveries). Hospitals with higher caesarean section rates (see Exhibit 17) can therefore expect higher overall lengths of stay. But average lengths of stay for the same type of delivery also vary twofold across the country.

'Trusts with higher than average lengths of stay should investigate the causes and, where possible, instigate appropriate remedies.'

115. Some of the variation is caused by differing administrative procedures in trusts. One example of this is the arrangements in place for baby checks. In many trusts, babies born in hospital are examined by paediatricians prior to discharge. In others, other professional groups (midwives and advanced neonatal nurse practitioners) are being trained to carry out these examinations. Policies on baby checks vary between trusts and can mean that discharge is delayed if women are waiting for paediatricians' ward rounds. There is a lack of consensus on the best arrangements for examining the newborn.

116. Trusts with higher than average lengths of stay should investigate the causes and, where possible, instigate appropriate remedies. For example, some trusts have made arrangements giving women easier access to paediatricians; for example, by providing a walk-in clinic at set times of day, so that mothers can take their babies for checking prior to hospital discharge.

117. However, care should be exercised in relation to lengths of stay. Women have different views about staying in hospital, and it is not clear that there is a 'right length' for first-time mothers, a different 'right length' for women who have had forceps deliveries, and so on. In the Audit Commission survey, the majority of women felt that their length of stay in hospital was 'about right', but 25 per cent were dissatisfied with it. While dissatisfaction is mainly associated with long lengths of stay (probably in part due to adverse delivery events) some women are being discharged from hospital before they feel ready.

118. It is essential that policies on length of stay are flexible. What matters most to women is being consulted about what happens to them. Women in the Audit Commission survey who felt that they 'had a say' in when they went home were almost twice as likely to be satisfied with their time in hospital. This included women who went home after a short stay as well as those whose stay was longer.

119. Reducing length of stay is seen as one way of relieving pressure on resources, and indeed some hospitals have reduced the number of postnatal beds substantially. But the extent of savings may be small. The days at the end of a stay have low marginal costs, so the cost savings will not be proportionate. Moreover, reducing hospital stays could increase the amount of care required from community services. On the other hand, reducing the length of stay and the number of women on the ward can mean that there is an opportunity to improve the quality of care that is provided, by freeing up some staff time.

Hospital staffing levels

120. Midwifery staffing levels and workloads on postnatal wards (and combined antenatal and postnatal wards) varied more than threefold between the trusts visited. This can happen for a variety of reasons:

◆ antenatal inpatient activity on postnatal wards accounts for between 10 per cent and 40 per cent of admissions in the trusts visited (the needs of antenatal patients also vary widely in themselves). Some wards do no antenatal work, while others provide antenatal day assessment and early labour assessment as well as caring for women who need inpatient care antenatally;

◆ the boundary between what is done by staff on postnatal wards versus neonatal units (NNUs) in relation to the care of babies needing special care differs from trust to trust (Exhibit 20);

◆ the extent to which support staff are employed on the wards, in addition to qualified midwives, also affects workload;

◆ the extent to which midwives on these wards act as a stand-by resource for the labour ward influences staffing levels; and

◆ the way midwifery care is organised. In some trusts, staffing ratios vary widely because there are set staffing levels regardless of the workload. In others – for example, where there is team midwifery – there may be a core of staff on the ward, working alongside 'team' midwives who come and go according to the needs of women on their caseload.

121. Differences in the type of care that postnatal wards provide and in the way that trusts staff the wards make it hard to reach a judgement on appropriate staffing levels. In some trusts, it is not uncommon to have only one midwife on duty on the postnatal ward (for example, at night), and certainly staff in many maternity units consider postnatal ward staffing to be too low. Trusts need to clarify what they are aiming to achieve in postnatal care in hospital, develop standards for quality of care (supporting breastfeeding, for example) and review the skills required. Once they have done this, they can determine the number and mix of staff that they need to staff the wards efficiently. Trusts can also aim to staff flexibly: they may, for example, review bookings and plan for predictably busy or quiet periods.

122. Trusts need to respond to concerns about staffing. For example, some trusts have had particular problems staffing postnatal wards in conjunction with a system of team midwifery (in which team midwives come into hospital to see 'their' women on the wards). Sometimes responsibilities are unclear, and a recent evaluation of one such scheme found tension between 'hospital' and 'team' midwives working alongside each other on the postnatal ward. Managers need to be aware of these issues and take steps to clarify roles, and ensure that core staff are not undervalued (Ref.19).

Exhibit 20
The care of babies on postnatal wards

The boundary between the postnatal ward and the neonatal unit differs from trust to trust.

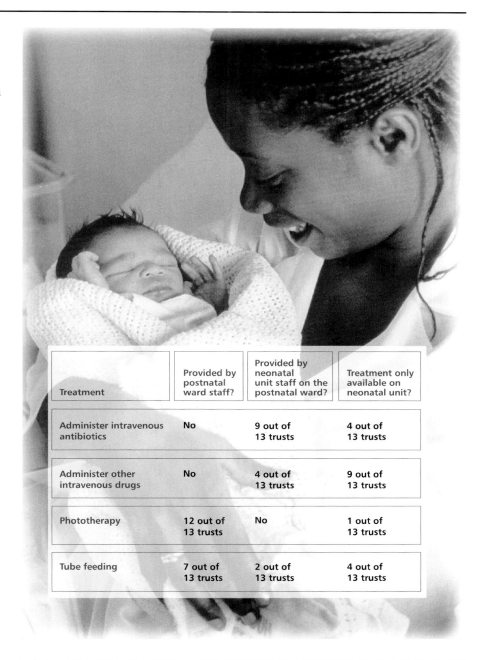

Treatment	Provided by postnatal ward staff?	Provided by neonatal unit staff on the postnatal ward?	Treatment only available on neonatal unit?
Administer intravenous antibiotics	No	9 out of 13 trusts	4 out of 13 trusts
Administer other intravenous drugs	No	4 out of 13 trusts	9 out of 13 trusts
Phototherapy	12 out of 13 trusts	No	1 out of 13 trusts
Tube feeding	7 out of 13 trusts	2 out of 13 trusts	4 out of 13 trusts

Source: Audit Commission study sites

123. Some trusts have responded to particular areas of concern. For example, in one trust staff were particularly concerned about the special care of babies on postnatal wards. In response to this, they actively involved NNU staff in the training and support of staff on the postnatal ward and in the production of clinical guidelines. Following this initiative, both NNU and postnatal staff felt more satisfied with the quality of care, and more confident about the special care of babies.

Home visiting by midwives

124. Postnatal home visits are popular with most women. However, their purpose is largely unspecified, and there is no evidence as to their clinical effectiveness including, for example, the effect on breastfeeding rates. Some women may require daily (or more frequent) visits if, for example, they are having problems establishing breastfeeding. Other women, especially those who already have children, may not need to see the midwife very often. Many women recognise this, and one in five say that the frequency of visits is not right for them.

125. The usual practice of visiting all women every day for the first few days following birth should be re-evaluated. One possibility would be to introduce some form of targeting. But in the absence of guidelines, this would depend on individual midwives' judgements, and runs the risk of those in most need (who present the greatest challenge to professionals) receiving less than appropriate care. Some trusts have addressed these issues by increasing the management focus and clinical leadership of midwifery teams, focusing in particular on issues including the targeting of midwives' home visits (Case Study 3).

Case Study 3
Targeting midwives' work on postnatal home visits

Scunthorpe and Goole Hospitals NHS Trust

All the midwives employed by Scunthorpe and Goole Hospitals NHS Trust are organised into nine teams delivering all antenatal care, care in labour and delivery and some postnatal care. (Although hospital postnatal care is planned by these teams, it is largely provided by hospital core staff.)

Each team is managed by a leader who is also a practising midwife member of the team. She organises the workload and on-call rotas, co-ordinates the midwives in her team and supervises junior midwives.

The head of the service uses the information collected by the midwives to target their work and assess their clinical practice. This information includes:

- the number and location of antenatal checks;
- the number and type of deliveries;
- whether the midwife or an obstetrician carried out the delivery;
- details about deliveries (eg, type of delivery, APGAR score, whether an episiotomy was carried out); and
- the number of postnatal visits.

Introducing priorities for midwives' work and reviewing the number of postnatal visits by teams showed that one team was doing a lot more visiting than the others. On investigation, the additional visits were found to be for breastfeeding advice. Since this was a rural team and home visits to women involved a great deal of travelling, the trust is now considering a postnatal clinic in the area, so that women can come to the midwives instead. This would reduce the amount of time that the midwives spend on postnatal visiting and travel while still meeting the needs of the women.

126. Trusts need to produce local guidelines (based on clear criteria and the best available evidence) for targeting home visiting. This means setting priorities so that care is directed at those most in need. They should specify the purpose of visits. The NHS Research and Development Initiative is supporting a number of research studies which will contribute evidence on effective practice in home visiting and the appropriate role of support workers. As research evidence accumulates about the most effective means of providing these services, it should be incorporated into local guidelines and practice. It is essential that the use of such guidelines is monitored. Postnatal depression is an area which needs particular research into the most effective care that can be provided.

127. There are clearly potential trade-offs between hospital and home care. Reducing length of hospital stay may mean greater demand for home visits, but in the long term it would probably still cost less overall. The average staffing cost of a postnatal visit (less than £10) is considerably less than a day as an inpatient (around £100 on average) (Ref. 61). Much will depend on the size of the shift and the ability of hospitals to reduce staff numbers in the hospital setting as a consequence.

The quality of postnatal care

Hospital facilities

128. Whatever balance of hospital and community care is chosen, it is important that the environment in hospital is reasonably good. Facilities on the postnatal ward can contribute to the recovery of mothers from the birth experience and their overall sense of well-being. Safety and security, quality of food and privacy for feeding are all important. The availability of clean baths, showers, and toilets also matters. Special facilities are needed for families whose baby has died, is unwell or disabled, or has other problems.

129. Many women value the provision of a 'debriefing' facility which enables them to review labour and birth events with a professional who is familiar with their care (Refs. 20, 21).

130. In some trusts the ward environments are poor, with only a few cramped bathrooms and inadequate eating areas. Women remark on poor food and hygiene. Apart from measures to improve security, upgrading of postnatal facilities is generally assigned a low priority. When prioritising competing demands on hospital resources, it is important for trusts to remember the impact that poor facilities can have on women's recollection of their experience, and on whether they will want to use the hospital again for later pregnancies.

> *'Of 13 trusts visited, only eight could provide information on breastfeeding rates on transfer from hospital to community services.'*

Infant feeding

131. One aspect of postnatal care that is known to promote both maternal and child health is encouraging and supporting women in breastfeeding. Breastfed babies are less likely to get gastroenteritis, asthma and respiratory diseases. It is also said to help establish good mother/baby relationships, and it is cheaper, both for mothers and the NHS. For families where infant formulas are the chosen or necessary method of feeding, information and support are equally important.

132. Interest in promoting breastfeeding has been given new impetus by the World Health Organisation's 'Baby Friendly Initiative' which aims to encourage all women to feed their babies exclusively on breast milk for the first four months. Hospitals can apply for 'baby friendly status' under an accreditation scheme.

133. Despite this high policy priority, breastfeeding rates in the UK do not appear to be changing and in some subgroups of the population, they are declining (Ref. 62). The Audit Commission survey showed that 68 per cent of women breastfed their babies at some stage and that 30 per cent were still breastfeeding when their babies were three months old. Of 13 trusts visited, only eight could provide information on breastfeeding rates on transfer from hospital to community services.

134. Trusts have an important part to play in promoting breastfeeding through the way that they organise postnatal care. As first steps, they need to establish a breastfeeding policy and to monitor breastfeeding rates – both initially and on discharge from midwifery services. They need to ensure that staff are trained to give sound and consistent advice on all aspects of infant feeding. Alternative means of providing breastfeeding support could be considered. For example, some trusts were in discussions with local breastfeeding counsellors and were hoping to involve them more on postnatal wards. Others had established a specialist role and training for breastfeeding advisers.

Care of sick babies in neonatal units

135. NNUs provide a range of services, from 24-hour emergency resuscitation of the newborn, through special care to intensive care, including assisted ventilation. A proportion of babies, depending on the unit, will require transfer to a more specialist centre (Refs. 63, 64) and either the referring or the receiving unit will provide clinical support for the transfer. Some NNUs also care for well babies whose mothers are seriously ill. Approximately 10 per cent of newborn babies are admitted to a NNU (Exhibit 21).

Exhibit 21
Neonatal unit admission rates

Variable admission rates are due to differences in types of unit, case-mix and current local practices.

Percentage of deliveries

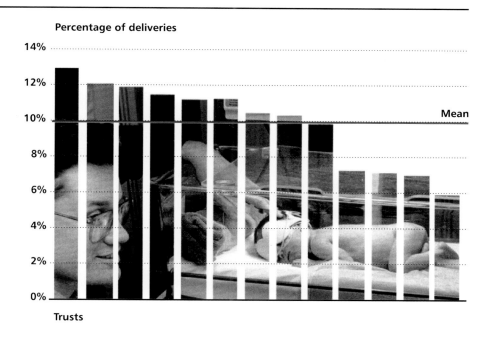

Trusts

Source: Audit Commission study sites

136. Although the average dependency of babies in NNUs is increasing, largely because of improving survival of low birthweight and pre-term infants, there is a wide range of clinical problems and levels of dependency within any neonatal unit (Ref. 65). Twins and higher order multiple pregnancies are also more likely to lead to pre-term births and neonatal unit admissions, and their numbers have increased markedly over the last decade (Ref. 66).

137. Three aspects of NNUs merit particular attention:

♦   activity;

♦   staffing; and

♦   parental support.

Activity

138. Neonatal units differ in their size and in the dependency of the babies they treat, with a more than fourfold variation in the scale of intensive care activity at the trusts visited. These differences are partly to do with the type of unit (for example, some trusts have more specialised skills and receive transfers of pregnant women whose babies are expected to need NNU admission). However, they are also due to historical factors (local support, expertise and enthusiasm), current practices (including different thresholds for admission) and the quality of care and skills available on the postnatal ward (for example, for babies requiring observation). Some trusts have

'In the long term, purchasers need to plan the extent to which NNU provision will be concentrated in more specialised larger regional centres as opposed to smaller, more local units.'

established transitional care wards where babies who might otherwise need admission to a NNU (for example, for observation) can be cared for alongside their mothers. In smaller trusts, where the viability of the unit has been questioned, there can be an incentive to admit babies to the NNU, in order to show a clear demand for local services.

139. Low levels of activity in neonatal care are important for two main reasons. Firstly, clinicians believe that a minimum level of activity is necessary for staff to maintain adequate skills, particularly for more intensive care. The minimum proposed (500 intensive care days per year) is thought sufficient to ensure adequate skills among medical and nursing staff to provide a continuing neonatal service, beyond initial resuscitation and stabilisation of babies (Ref. 67). Secondly, low thresholds for admission may well be traumatic for families and wasteful of resources. For these reasons, admission rates to NNUs should be closely monitored and subject to multidisciplinary audit.

140. Further research is needed on the relationship between the degree of specialisation and outcomes for babies. However, where units do not have sufficient skills and experience to provide highly specialised care, there is clearly a need for rationalisation that is jointly planned by purchasers and trusts. Planning is made more difficult by a lack of information on the volume of NNU activity (and particularly on intensive care activity). Although all units should routinely record overall levels of activity and intensive care days, four of 13 NNUs visited were unable to quantify their intensive care activity. These basic data should be mandatory and insisted upon by purchasers.

141. In the long term, purchasers need to plan the extent to which NNU provision will be concentrated in more specialised larger regional centres as opposed to smaller, more local units. There are benefits and drawbacks to each (Exhibit 22). An initiative in Wales has already focused attention and funding on a review of the balance between regional and small units (Refs. 68, 69). In the short term, units need to make efforts to address the drawbacks and ensure that transport arrangements are good.

142. An approach that is being tried in one region has been to propose a differential referral strategy: babies likely to be born before 26 weeks gestation are delivered in one of the larger maternity units in the region, following in utero transfer (Ref. 70). At the same time, it is being proposed that large district hospitals, presently undertaking neonatal intensive care, should accept greater numbers of inward transfers of more mature babies who require such care. If there is to be collaboration of this sort, neonatal transfers should be undertaken only by skilled, experienced and well-equipped transport teams (Ref. 64).

Exhibit 22
Providing neonatal care in larger regional and smaller local units

There are benefits and risks to both regional and local provision.

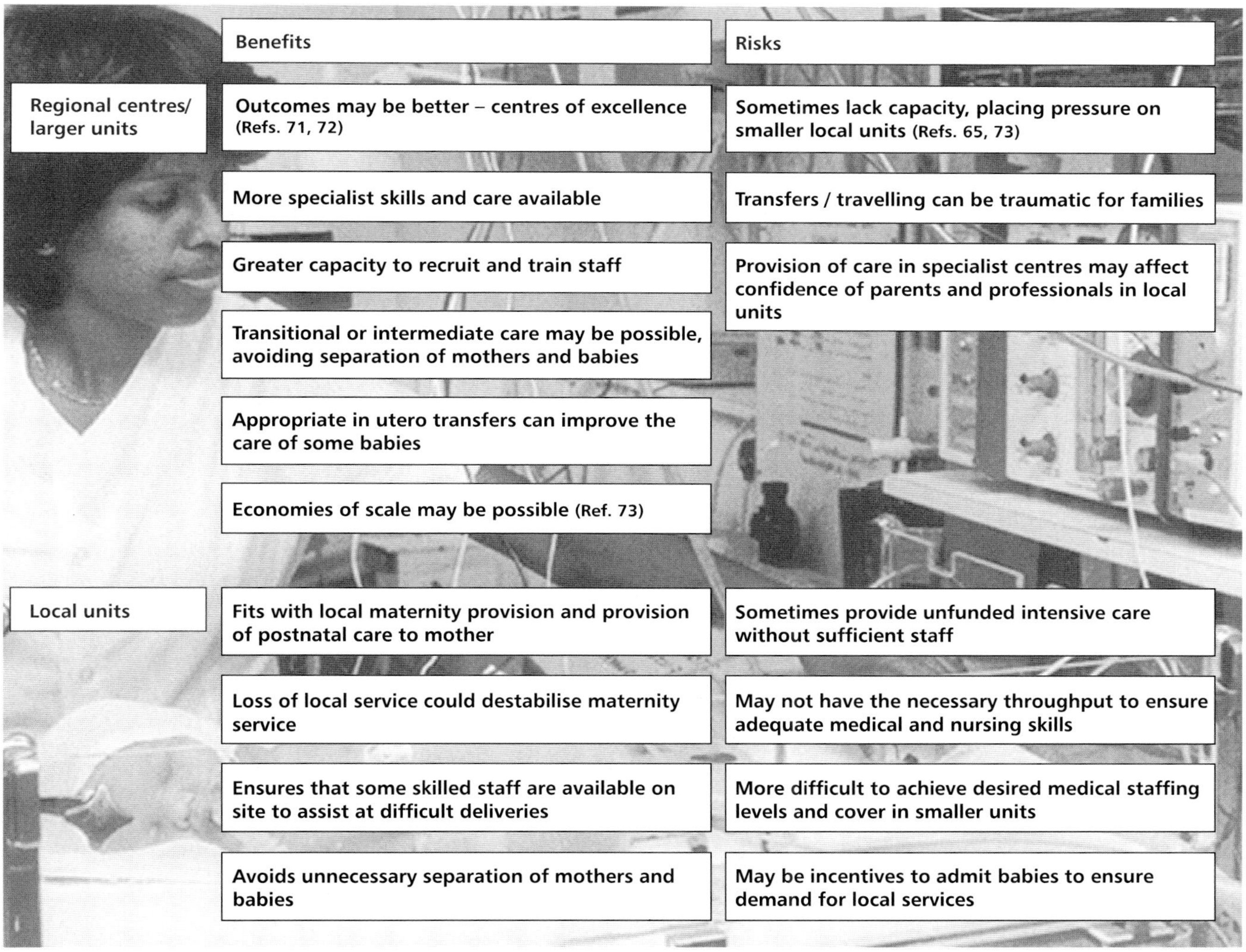

	Benefits	Risks
Regional centres/ larger units	Outcomes may be better – centres of excellence (Refs. 71, 72)	Sometimes lack capacity, placing pressure on smaller local units (Refs. 65, 73)
	More specialist skills and care available	Transfers / travelling can be traumatic for families
	Greater capacity to recruit and train staff	Provision of care in specialist centres may affect confidence of parents and professionals in local units
	Transitional or intermediate care may be possible, avoiding separation of mothers and babies	
	Appropriate in utero transfers can improve the care of some babies	
	Economies of scale may be possible (Ref. 73)	
Local units	Fits with local maternity provision and provision of postnatal care to mother	Sometimes provide unfunded intensive care without sufficient staff
	Loss of local service could destabilise maternity service	May not have the necessary throughput to ensure adequate medical and nursing skills
	Ensures that some skilled staff are available on site to assist at difficult deliveries	More difficult to achieve desired medical staffing levels and cover in smaller units
	Avoids unnecessary separation of mothers and babies	May be incentives to admit babies to ensure demand for local services

Source: Audit Commission

Staffing

143. Given the variations in activity of NNUs, it is not surprising that staffing levels also vary substantially. The number of qualified nurses per cot, for example, varied threefold at the trusts visited (Exhibit 23). Some units have more difficulty than others in recruiting and retaining skilled staff.

144. In some cases, low neonatal unit staffing levels reflect difficulty with recruitment and retention: almost all of the units visited had vacancies and annual turnover varied substantially (from 0–14 per cent). Faced with these difficulties, some units are operating all their official cots and more besides, but with inadequate nursing levels, while others are deliberately keeping some cots empty.

145. The wide fluctuations in demand for neonatal care mean that staff may come under pressure from time to time. Managers have a variety of possible solutions available to them both in the short and long term. In the short term, staffing arrangements can be altered – for example, with present staff working extra or longer shifts, borrowing staff from other departments or employing bank or agency staff. These solutions can help in the short term, but may have consequences for staff morale or for the quality of care, if unknown or unqualified staff are used. As an alternative, managers can change short-term activity levels. This can mean that units close or refuse admissions, with the consequent effects on families if babies have to be

Exhibit 23
Neonatal unit staffing

There is a threefold variation in the number of qualified nurses per cot.

*Cot numbers adjusted as follows: special care cots were counted as 1, and intensive care cots were counted as 5.5 to reflect the dependency of the babies and therefore the case-mix of different units. This is in accordance with current recommended staffing levels for intensive care and special care babies (Ref. 74).

Source: Audit Commission study sites

Nurses per cot*

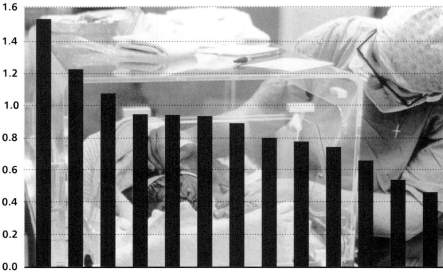

Trusts

transferred elsewhere. In the longer term, the staffing establishment can be reviewed alongside the number and type of cots. Whatever the local solution chosen, better planning at regional level and taking a longer term view are key.

146. Some small units are also finding it difficult to provide medical cover to the required standards because they are short of doctors. Recent increases in the number of junior medical staff have improved the situation, allowing reduced on-call and the operation of full or partial shift systems (Ref. 75). All the trusts visited with more than 4,000 deliveries per year had dedicated senior house officers working in neonatal care and, with the introduction of new posts, middle-grade cover was adequate in these larger units. However, in the units with fewer than 4,000 deliveries per year medical staffing problems are still evident.

147. Units do not just differ in the number of staff they employ: levels of skill also vary. A recent national survey found that 44 per cent of neonatal nursing staff had a post-registration qualification in the specialty (Ref. 75), compared to the 70 per cent level currently recommended (Ref. 76): a level reached by only two of the trusts visited. Furthermore, there has been some concern about staff who are qualified neither as nurses nor midwives caring for babies on NNUs (Ref. 75). The proportion of unqualified staff, usually nursery nurses and nursing auxiliaries, varied considerably between units (from 10–38 per cent of staff).

148. Despite concerns about unqualified staff, and the fact that some NNUs have a policy of reducing their role in direct care, most units continue to employ them. In some cases they have made great efforts to provide additional training for these staff so that they can become qualified. While this is a welcome initiative, there are concerns about the transferability of local training 'certificates'. Once again, regional planning is needed to ensure that trusts collaborate to ensure that such training is transferable.

149. Some trusts have relieved the pressure on medical staff by recruiting and training advanced neonatal nurse practitioners, a development that was popular at the trusts visited. They are a relatively recent development in the UK, with nationally recognised courses and qualifications. Following an intensive training course and consolidation of their role and skills, they are able not only to attend to the medical and nursing needs of NNU patients, but also to act as a resource for teaching colleagues. They are able to attend difficult deliveries on the labour ward and in theatre, examine babies on the postnatal ward and relieve the intensity of work for junior medical staff. In some units they participate in the junior doctors' rota and many are involved in training such staff, particularly at the time of their introduction and orientation to the unit (Ref. 77).

Parental support

150. Parents of babies in NNUs need good support, information and practical help (Ref. 75). Many wish to participate in their baby's care and all need to be kept informed about the care and condition of their baby. And mothers may have their own health needs at this time.

151. These special requirements are not always well handled by units whose prime role is, after all, to focus on the needs of the baby. One in six mothers of NNU babies in the Commission's survey had problems in visiting their baby: in some cases overnight accommodation may not be available, and parents are not always welcomed or involved (Exhibit 24).

152. The variable quality and nature of the information and facilities available does not help. Not all units had information booklets explaining the equipment or giving guidance on hygiene procedures, and relatively few gave parents written information and advice about discharge and taking their baby home.

153. Trusts should review their facilities for parents and the extent to which they are used. Referral centres need to pay particular attention to this: each large unit should ideally have several rooms for parents to stay overnight. These should be separate from rooms used by junior medical staff. Parents whose babies have been cared for in the unit in the past can be a valuable source of information for trusts on the ways in which facilities can be improved.

154. Some developments, such as the provision of a private area for breastfeeding, do not require significant extra resource but a reorganisation of existing facilities, and a clear message from staff that their efforts are supported. Other areas will require ongoing innovation and evaluation. And lastly, trusts must recognise the vital role that parents play in the care of their babies and give them practical help and support.

Exhibit 24
Some mothers felt that they were not fully involved in their baby's care

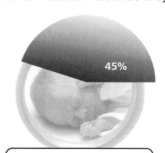
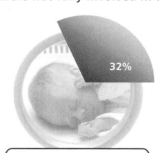
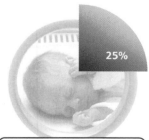
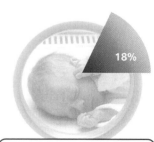

45%	32%	25%	18%
...felt that they could not always have the people to visit that they wanted	...felt that they could not always stay with their baby during the doctors' ward round	...did not always feel included in their baby's care	...did not always feel that they could be with their baby as long as they wanted

Source: Audit Commission – survey of recent mothers

Recommendations

Postnatal care

Clinicians and managers in trusts should:

1   involve women in decisions about how long they will stay in hospital and the pattern of postnatal care that they will receive at home.

2   clarify the objectives and set standards for postnatal care in hospital and at home.

3   review staffing and the skill mix required to meet these objectives.

4   promote breastfeeding and monitor breastfeeding rates initially and at the time of discharge from the care of community midwives. This may require investment in the training of breastfeeding support workers.

5   develop guidelines for matching home visiting to the needs of mothers and their families.

6   compare the average lengths of hospital stay for women experiencing each type of delivery with those in other trusts, and investigate and remove administrative procedures that prolong lengths of stay.

The NHS Executive should:

7   prioritise research into effective postnatal care for mothers and babies to help the service develop cost-effective postnatal care

Care of sick babies in neonatal units

Clinicians and managers in trusts should:

8   review staffing levels and skill-mix, and consider recruiting and training neonatal nurse practitioners.

9   review activity levels. Where these are insufficient to sustain adequate medical and nursing skills, trusts should consider stopping the provision of long-term specialist intensive care services.

10   review admission policies and arrangements for the care of babies with minor problems or for those requiring observation only.

11   make sure that parents are made welcome by staff in NNUs and that arrangements are in place to provide them with information, access and practical support (such as overnight accommodation). Parents whose babies have previously been cared for in NNUs can help to pinpoint areas where quality can be improved.

12   assess relationships and links with neighbouring units, taking a more co-ordinated approach to this aspect of care.

Commissioners should:

13   plan services on a geographical basis, and ensure that the activity purchased is within safe levels, and includes the planning of transport arrangements.

14   define the data set they require trusts to collect on neonatal activity (including intensive care days) along with a clear requirement for the ongoing audit of admission rates.

15   utilise the British Paediatric Association (BPA)/British Association of Perinatal Medicine (BAPM) standards in the contracting process.

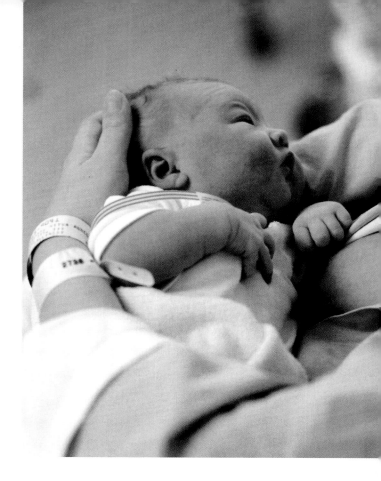

5 The Way Forward

The challenge for the NHS is to continue to meet high expectations of services while making sure that the best use of resources is being made and that services are clinically effective. Women need to be listened to and involved in decisions. Women whose experience of pregnancy and childbirth is for whatever reason difficult or disappointing need special consideration.

Health authorities can improve information about local services. Clinicians and managers in trusts should work together to improve communication. Clinical guidelines and protocols can improve continuity and consistency in information and the way that it is provided.

The pressure on trusts to do more for less – to keep pace with expectations, increase activity and deliver safe, clinically effective care at less cost – will not go away. Purchasers and trusts must ensure that resources are used as efficiently as possible, establish a clear sense of direction for the service as a whole, and cost planned changes so that they can prioritise competing demands for action.

Introduction

155. Current policy in England and Wales has set the agenda for maternity services. As the NHS looks forward to maternity care in the next century, the challenge will be to continue to meet users' justifiably high expectations of services. In order to meet this challenge, managers and clinicians will need to be sure they are making the very best use of their resources and delivering clinically effective care. This chapter draws together the issues for the service as a whole and considers the way forward.

Variations in patterns of care

156. The variation in services that characterises maternity care would not be a problem if it reflected differences in case-mix or in what local women want. However, there is no convincing evidence that this is the case. The quality of data makes it difficult to assess case-mix, and mothers report that they are not always given much choice about the type of care that they receive. It seems likely that much of the variation is simply the result of history.

157. The solution to variation, however, is not standardisation. It is for purchasers to determine priorities and actively to shape local services. Health authorities are charged with the responsibility for investigating local women's views, involving GPs in strategy and improving the effectiveness of clinical care (Refs. 78 - 81). The extent to which they are investigating local views varies: only one of the 12 authorities surveyed by the Audit Commission had achieved good guidance from the local population about the changes needed in maternity services. Most authorities could make better use of the expertise of the Maternity Services Liaison Committee (MSLC) and involve local providers (trusts and GPs) more in strategic decisions. Guidance recently produced for MSLCs should help to strengthen their role (Ref. 82).

158. Some health authorities have funded *Changing Childbirth* projects, the majority of which are pilot team and caseload midwifery projects. Comparatively few have brought about change in the main body of the service: eight of the 12 authorities did not have a strategy for maternity services as a whole; six included maternity care in large block contracts either for 'acute' or for 'women's' services. The degree to which the contracts were specified varied.

159. In the absence of a clear lead from purchasers, trusts – and sometimes individual clinicians within trusts – have taken responsibility for key decisions about services, such as what antenatal screening and testing services they will provide or the extent to which they will involve GPs in shared care protocols. Health authorities must take responsibility for decisions about the levels and types of service that they commission and improve the specifications in contracts (Case Study 4).

Case Study 4
Commissioning maternity services

Southern Derbyshire Health Authority

Southern Derbyshire Health Authority developed its strategy for maternity services in collaboration with its local provider. It started by consulting local women in 1991 through a validated questionnaire survey.

The strategy, completed in 1994, set one main objective for maternity services: 'by the year 2000 maximum health gain should be obtained for childbearing women through a cost-effective women-and family-centred service based on sound clinical practice'.

This objective translates into 11 key targets, four of which relate to clinical matters, three to service delivery and four to organisational matters. These expand into subtargets, with essential and proposed actions, which form the basis for service specifications.

For example: the target for breastfeeding reads: 'Every woman should receive full and consistent advice on feeding, whichever method she chooses, by 1996.' An essential action following this was that purchasers agreed common guidelines for infant feeding to be applied by all providers. This has led to the Southern Derbyshire breastfeeding policy.

The health authority monitors performance against strategy by asking providers for outcomes on:

◆ type of delivery;

◆ stillbirths and infant mortality/morbidity;

◆ selected factors associated with adverse outcomes;

◆ maternal morbidity;

◆ selected aspects of service provision;

◆ evidence of effective auditing systems;

◆ data from surveys of women;

◆ *Changing Childbirth*; and

◆ breastfeeding.

An annual specification based on the strategy is agreed as part of the contractual arrangements with the local provider. The strategy is reviewed regularly.

Fragmentation

160. Variation is not a problem in itself if it reflects differing needs, but fragmentation of service delivery is a problem. It can occur with shared care, or because women move between trusts for different aspects of their care, and is often made worse by poor communication. Whatever the cause, fragmentation reduces the capacity of the service as a whole to bring about beneficial change, jeopardises continuity, makes woman-centred care harder to achieve and frustrates professional and support staff.

161. Purchasers can help to mitigate the effects: they can bring GPs and specialists together to plan maternity and neonatal services; and promote joint protocols, clinical guidelines and joint audit. Securing GPs' involvement in decisions about service plans and delivery is crucial. Around 45 per cent of those surveyed by the Commission reported that GPs in their local area had been involved in developing clinical guidelines, referral criteria and patterns of maternity care.

162. Trusts can make sure that GPs are equipped with accurate and up-to-date information about their services, and that the communication with GPs works well. Trusts that deliver highly specialised care to women and babies must take particular care to communicate with other trusts that are also caring for the same women and families. Where separate departments in the same trust are involved in maternity care, it is up to clinical directors and managers to make sure that services are planned and delivered around the women's needs and not their own. The larger the organisation the more difficult, and the more important, it will be to bring all the various parties together. Hand-held records and the national standard maternity record currently in development will help, but it will always be important to consult staff widely.

Woman-centred services: information and choice

163. *Changing Childbirth* has succeeded in raising awareness of pregnant women's needs for information, and the importance of listening to their views and involving them in decisions about their care. It is impossible to overestimate the value that pregnant women place on information about their own and their babies' well-being, and there is always more that can be done. Some women feel better informed and more in control of key aspects of their care than others. Women whose experience of pregnancy and motherhood is – for whatever reason – difficult, disappointing, or out of line with the common expectations, need special consideration.

164. Some health authorities have made comprehensive, up-to-date and detailed information about local services available to women through GP surgeries and other outlets (Ref. 83). Funding was also recently given to the NHS Centre for Reviews and Dissemination from the NHS Executive for the development of evidence-based information such as that recently produced by MIDIRS (Ref. 33).

165. In trusts, clinicians and managers should work together to improve communication, especially in antenatal screening and testing which is known to present problems for staff as well as to women using the service. If staff need help and training in communication and communication skills, trusts should provide it. Clinical guidelines and protocols can improve continuity and consistency in information-giving, and a common maternity record will make it easier for clinicians to see what others are doing. As new evidence becomes available that challenges established practices, purchasers,

'It is especially important that clinicians enter into public debates about the objectives for services and the reasons for change.'

providers and clinicians must take collective responsibility for educating women and the general public and for explaining the rationales behind the service that is being provided.

166. In some areas, managers and clinicians are concerned that the emphasis on woman-centredness might conflict with service objectives. They question, for example, whether reducing the pattern of antenatal care for women at low risk of complications is compatible with giving women what they want. And what should the obstetrician do when he or she is asked to do a caesarean section that is not justified clinically? As yet, there is no conclusive evidence that supports a move in any direction, but questions about the relationship between choice and other service objectives will not go away.

167. Managers and clinicians are responsible for making the best and most equitable use of the resources available on behalf of the local population. There may be circumstances in which they are not able to meet an individual's expectation and still fulfil their obligations to the community as a whole. They may, for example, have to use their authority to explain the rationale behind a reduced pattern of antenatal care for women at low risk of complications in pregnancy, and to explain to women and the public at large the thinking behind their priorities. It is especially important that clinicians enter into public debates about the objectives for services and the reasons for change. When and if conflicts arise between service objectives, they need support from their managers and from the purchasers in putting forward policies that promote efficiency and effectiveness. Within this kind of policy framework, clinicians should also be free to consider each individual case on its own merits.

Improving efficiency

168. The pressure on trusts to do more for less – to keep pace with expectations, increase activity and deliver safe, clinically effective care at less cost – will not go away. Purchasers and trusts must ensure that resources are used as efficiently as possible.

169. Health authorities need to make sure that contracts are more specific. They should discourage duplication between trusts and GPs and target specialist care on the women who need it most. Health authorities and trusts need more systematic information about patterns of care and case-mix and they should collaborate to collect it.

170. The first priority for both purchasers and trusts should be to improve mainstream maternity services. They need a clear sense of direction for the service as a whole and a coherent view on where their 'pilot' projects fit in. It is essential to cost planned changes in the organisation of maternity care so that they can choose between competing priorities.

Effective care

171. As a first step in tackling variations in practice, the quality of routinely collected data needs to be improved. The NHS Executive has an important role in specifying the data to be collected and guiding purchasers and trusts. The collection of key indicators which take case-mix into account should be prioritised.

172. Obstetrics was the first specialty to have access to systematic reviews of evidence (via the Cochrane database)(Ref. 10), and the focus on evidence-based practice is well-developed. There is still a need for more and better evidence on some aspects of service provision. An improved focus on evidence needs to be grounded in a culture which accepts that evidence changes and practice should change to reflect it.

173. But there is also a need to pay more attention to bringing the evidence that does exist into clinical practice. Systematic reviews are not well disseminated, with 72 per cent of trusts recently surveyed not having access to the database of clinical trials in maternity care (Ref. 84), although progress is being made in this area (Ref. 34). Eighty per cent of GPs surveyed by the Commission said they did not have access to the Cochrane database.

174. Both purchasers and trusts need to prioritise systematic, multidisciplinary audit and should include audit requirements and key indicators in service specifications. Trusts must take steps to disseminate evidence on effective care (for a start, making the Cochrane database available and easily accessible to all clinical staff) as well as taking other steps to change practice.

Conclusions

175. Maternity services are facing great change. This report has highlighted some areas of service that should be the focus for improvement, within which purchasers and trusts should prioritise key areas for action. Despite their generally positive views, staff surveyed at the trusts visited expressed concerns about the demands made of them: about their workload, skills and responsibilities, and the environment in which they work. There are also areas of service provision where improvements are possible in both the effectiveness and efficiency of services. These are factors that need to be considered alongside women's views.

176. The emphasis in policy on service users is welcome but many of the changes currently taking place are at the margins. The effectiveness agenda is an important part of the policy which must now be prioritised for action. There is a need for strong leadership to bring about the changes required at the core of the service for all women.

177. This report summarises the key points for action. It will be followed by local audits of maternity services in every trust in England and Wales in 1997 carried out by the Commission's auditors. These will identify the issues in the local context, and assist professionals locally in developing a plan for action.

Recommendations

Trusts should:

1 make sure that clinicians have access to systematic reviews of effectiveness and encourage the development of clinical guidelines and protocols.

2 improve information for women and their partners, especially in antenatal screening and testing.

Commissioners should:

3 actively involve women who use local maternity services and health professionals in helping to determine priorities.

4 work closely with GPs, trusts and neighbouring authorities to plan maternity and neonatal services.

5 use contracts to develop local services that deliver high quality, clinically effective care to women and babies, and that use resources efficiently.

6 base decisions about priorities on information about local users' views and experiences, as well as on costs.

The NHS Executive should:

7 support research into organisational as well as clinical apects of maternity care, including postnatal care, where there continues to be uncertainty.

8 assist purchasers and trusts in disseminating evidence-based information for professionals and service users.

9 provide support for measures that will improve the national data on maternity care, including key indicators of case-mix.

Appendix 1: Data Sources and Research Methods

1. Fieldwork at NHS Trusts

The study team visited 13 trusts in detail ('study sites') to gather data about maternity services. Two trusts were teaching hospitals and 11 were non-teaching. The study sites were selected so that there was a mix of:

◆ size (number of deliveries); and

◆ geographical spread and mix of urban and rural areas.

Table 1
Characteristics of study sites

Geographical spread		Size	
Region	Number of trusts visited	Number of deliveries per annum	Number of trusts visited
North/North East	3	< 2,000	3
North West	2	2,001 – 4,000	6
Midlands	2	> 4,001	4
Wales	2		
South East	3		
South West	1		

Data was collected by direct enquiry of the trust and by carrying out a number of interviews and surveys. The following surveys were carried out at each study site:

◆ detailed survey of 10 antenatal clinics;

◆ survey of 200 births on the labour ward;

◆ survey of staffing and activity on the labour ward and the antenatal/postnatal ward(s) over a 14-day period;

◆ diary survey of 10 community midwives over a two-week period;

◆ survey of staffing and activity on the neonatal unit over a 14-day period; and

◆ a staff attitudes survey of 50 midwives and all medical staff.

In addition, a number of short visits were made to other trusts, to investigate specific aspects of the service or areas of good practice. The complete list of all trusts visited is given below.

Bridgend and District NHS Trust (Princess of Wales Hospital), Central Manchester Healthcare NHS Trust (St Mary's Hospital for Women and Children), Chelsea and Westminster Healthcare NHS Trust, City Hospitals Sunderland, Derby City General Hospital NHS Trust, East Cheshire NHS Trust, Glan Hafren NHS Trust, Gloucestershire Royal NHS Trust, Guy's and St Thomas's Hospital NHS Trust, Kingston Hospital NHS Trust, Leicester Royal Infirmary NHS Trust, Liverpool Women's Hospital NHS Trust, Mid Essex Hospitals NHS Trust, Milton Keynes General NHS Trust, North Staffordshire Hospital NHS Trust (City General, Stoke-on-Trent), Royal Berkshire and Battle Hospitals NHS Trust, Scunthorpe and Goole Hospitals NHS Trust, Winchester and Eastleigh Healthcare NHS Trust.

Thanks are due to the staff of these trusts who assisted with data collection and who spent time talking to the study team.

2. Health authorities

The study team interviewed staff from 12 health authorities about purchasing maternity services. A pro-forma of the areas to be covered was supplied in advance, and on the basis of this a semi-structured telephone interview was conducted. The health authority nominated the most appropriate interviewee on the basis of the interview pro-forma.

The health authorities surveyed were:

Berkshire Health Authority, Buckinghamshire Health Authority; Gloucestershire Health Authority, Gwent Health Authority, Lechyd Morgannwg Health/West Glamorgan Health Authority, Liverpool Health Authority, Manchester Health Authority, North and Mid Hampshire Health Authority, North Staffordshire Health Authority, South Cheshire Health Authority, Southern Derbyshire Health Authority, Sunderland Health Authority, South Humber Health Authority

3. GPs

The study team carried out a survey of 500 GPs in five FHSA areas (following an initial pilot of 100 GPs in one FHSA area). One hundred GPs were selected at random from each FHSA. The FHSAs were selected from the same geographical areas as the study sites and therefore represented the same mix of type of area. GPs received a questionnaire which asked about their role in maternity care, their views of midwifery services and their future plans in maternity care.

This work was done in collaboration with Dr Sarah Clement, Department of General Practice, United Medical and Dental Schools of Guy's and St Thomas's Hospitals, London SE1.

First Class Delivery
Improving Maternity Services in England and Wales

Respondent profile

Characteristics of GPs and practices in the sample

Table 2
Age

	Percentage
Under 30	0.3%
30 – 39	20.3%
40 – 49	35.5%
50 or over	43.8%

Table 3
List size of practice

Patients	Percentage
up to 3,000	13.4%
3,001 – 6,000	28.6%
6,001 – 9,000	28.3%
over 9,000	29.7%

Table 4
Fundholding/non-fundholding status

	Percentage
Fundholding	46.7%
Non-fundholding	53.3%

Note: The response rate was 61 per cent.

Table 5
Geographical status

	Percentage
Rural	12.2%
Semi-rural	31.8%
Urban	43.7%
Inner city	12.2%

4. Survey of recent mothers

The Survey was carried out by MORI's health research unit on behalf of the Audit Commission, and was run at MORI by Mark Speed (Director, Social Research) and Trinh Tu (Research Executive). Self-completion questionnaires were sent to a national sample of 3,570 women who had given birth in a period during June and July 1995 at 16–18 weeks post partum. The sample was drawn by the Office of Population Censuses and Surveys from its birth registers, and was cross-checked with the register of deaths to ensure that women and babies who had subsequently died were excluded from the sample.

The method of administration was the same for the whole population, and no efforts were made to boost the sample from any subgroup of the population.

The data collected in this survey is to be published in full later in 1997.

Both the Audit Commission study team and MORI are grateful to all the mothers who spent time completing the questionnaire.

Table 6
Survey of recent mothers: respondent profile

	Total sample population (%)	Respondents (%)
ALL	**3,570**	**2,375**
Age (mean age of respondents was 29 years)		
<20	6%	6%
21-25	20%	19%
26-30	34%	37%
31-35	28%	28%
36-40	10%	9%
>40	2%	1%
Social Class (OPCS classification – women's occupation) P=<0.001		
Prof/intermediate	20%	23%
Skilled non-manual	25%	29%
Skilled manual	5%	5%
Partly skilled	8%	8%
Unskilled	1%	1%
Armed Forces	*	*
Inadequately described	1%	*
Economically inactive	40%	33%
Region		
North	5%	5%
Yorks and Humberside	10%	10%
East Midlands	8%	8%
East Anglia	4%	5%
South East	38%	37%
South West	9%	10%
West Midlands	10%	10%
North West	11%	11%
Wales	5%	5%

Note: * denotes less than 1 per cent but greater than 0.5 per cent. Data may not total 100 per cent due to rounding.

Social class was allocated according to the woman's occupation. This compares to the following data for all women over 16 years in England in 1991. Allocation was made on the basis of occupation in the week preceding the 1991 Census. Those who were unemployed were allocated according to their most recently paid job, unless they had been unemployed for more than 10 years. Social class I and II 18 per cent; III (N) 24 per cent; III (M) 4 per cent; IV 10 per cent; V 4 per cent; economically inactive (excluding retired) 36 per cent; Other 3 per cent. Base 1,509,204. Source: *1991 Census*, 10 per cent sample, OPCS.

Age data compare to OPCS 1994 birth statistics as follows: number of maternities to women aged less than 20 – 6 per cent; 20-24 – 21 per cent; 25-29 – 34 per cent; 30-34 – 27 per cent; 35-39 – 9 per cent; 40 plus – 2 per cent. Base 659,126. Source: VS2 1994 birth statistics, OPCS.

Regional data compares to the following regions data for women aged 16-44 in 1994: North 6 per cent; Yorkshire and Humberside 10 per cent; East Midlands 8 per cent; East Anglia 4 per cent; South East 36 per cent; South West 9 per cent; West Midlands 10 per cent; North West 12 per cent; Wales 5 per cent. Base 10,430,000. Source: *Regional Trends* 31 (1996 edition) London, HMSO.

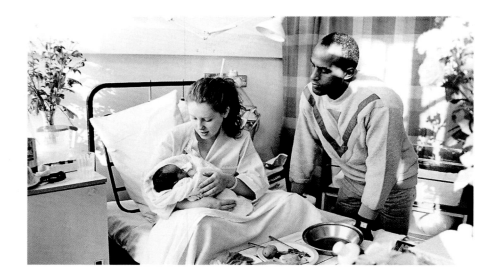

Table 7
Survey of recent mothers: summary statistics

Q	Percentage
Place of birth (base 2,375)	

Hospital	95%
Home	3%
GP unit	1%

Parity	First baby	42%
	Subsequent baby	58%

Intervention in labour (base 2,375)		
Induction		28%
Augmentation		52%
Mode of delivery	**Caesarean section (7.8 per cent planned CS)**	17%
	Forceps	6%
	Ventouse	5%
	Normal (vaginal)	70%

Admission of baby to a neonatal unit (base 2,211)	10%

Place of birth data compares to the following: Place of birth – hospital (NHS and other, incl GP units 98 per cent); home 2 per cent. Base 659,126. Source VS2 1994 birth statistics, OPCS.

Mode of delivery – These figures compare to the following rates in Hospital Episode System for England (1993/94). Spontaneous 73 per cent; forceps 7 per cent; ventouse 4 per cent; breech 1 per cent; caesarean (total) 15 per cent (elective caesarean 6 per cent). NB: these figures exclude deliveries where no method of delivery was recorded and those with no maternity HES record – approximately one-third of deliveries. Base number: 399,891.

Table 8
Survey of recent mothers: educational qualifications of respondents

Highest level of educational qualification (excluding professional qualifications) (base 2,375)	Audit Commission survey	General Household Survey 1993 (No. 24) (Women aged 16-39) Great Britain
None	12%	20%
GCSE/CSE/O level	41%	46%
A Level or higher	45%	32%
Not stated/other	2%	2%

Table 9
Survey of recent mothers: ethnic group

	Audit Commission Survey (base 2,284)	1991 Census data – women aged 15-44 percentage
White	93%	93%
Other ethnic groups combined (to give sufficient numbers for analysis)	6%	7%
Consisting of		
Black British	1%	Categorisation not used
Black Caribbean	1%	1%
Black African	1%	1%
Black other	*	*
Indian	1%	1%
Pakistani	1%	1%
Bangladeshi	*	*
Chinese	*	*
Not stated	1%	–
Other groups	2%	1%

Note: English was not the first language of 131 respondents (6 per cent).

Qualitative information

Among the 2,375 respondents were a substantial number of women (983) who made detailed comments about their care. These were coded and analysed in the categories shown below and according to whether they were positive or negative comments. Comments could relate to both the overall experience as well as the services received. Many women made a number of comments (528 made one comment, 455 made two or three comments), so analysis can be carried out as a proportion of women commenting, or by proportion of comments. A single comment could encompass up to three topics.

Comments were analysed by:

(i) Stage of care: antenatal, labour and delivery; postnatal (hospital or community); neonatal; or applied to the service as a whole.

ii) Theme or topic: (comments were first read to determine appropriate categories). The main categories were: communication; skill / care (including management of pain); information; continuity of care; choice; support; attitudes; organisation of care (eg, appointments systems).

(iii) The professional involved: GP, hospital doctor, midwife, unspecified hospital staff, neonatal staff, health visitors.

NB: The number of comments relating to particular professions is due in part to the amount of contact women have with them.

Table 10
Survey of recent mothers: summary of qualitative data

Antenatal	Labour	Postnatal	Neonatal	All phases	
115	95	86	8	192	**Positive**
301	269	443	12	38	**Negative**

Staff (unspecified)	GP	Hospital doctor	Midwife	Other	
120	32	33	257	36	**Positive**
27	107	144	613	73	**Negative**

Skill/care	Staff attitudes/ support	Organisation of services	Morbidity	Other themes combined	
284	97	4	4	97	**Positive**
189	217	115	95	431	**Negative**

Note: Totals are comments, not women. Most frequent areas for comment are shown – smaller categories are combined in 'other'.

Appendix 2: Advisory Group and Other Advisers

The study team is grateful for the guidance provided by the study Advisory Group and other advisers.

The advisory group

Ms Roxanne Chamberlain – National Childbirth Trust

Ms Jo Garcia – Social Scientist, National Perinatal Epidemiology Unit

Ms Kate Jackson – Director, Changing Childbirth Implementation Team, NHS Executive

Ms Kate Jenkins – Audit Commissioner

Ms Helen Lewison – National Childbirth Trust

Dr Mary Macintosh – Consultant Obstetrician, Institute of Epidemiology and Health Services Research and Leeds General Infirmary

Ms Beverley McLachlan – Senior Nurse Manager/Head of Midwifery, City General Hospital, Stoke-on-Trent

Ms Jane McKessack – Health Care Directorate, NHS Executive

Dr Maggie Redshaw – Research Psychologist, Department of Child Health, Royal Hospital for Sick Children, Bristol

Ms Hilary Rowland – Audit Commissioner

Ms Louise Silverton – Director of Education, Practice and Development, Royal College of Midwives

Ms Angela Sealey – Chairman, North and Mid Hampshire Health Commission

Mrs Helena Shovelton – Audit Commissioner

Dr Lindsay Smith – General Practitioner (nominated by the Royal College of General Practitioners)

Dr Luke Zander – General Practitioner

Additional advice was provided by:

Ms Soo Downe – Research midwife, Derby City General Hospital

Ms Miranda Mugford – Health economist, National Perinatal Epidemiology Unit

Dr Richard Johansen – Consultant obstetrician, City General Hospital, Stoke-on-Trent

Dr Geoffrey Chamberlain – Consultant obstetrician, Singleton Hospital, Swansea

Dr Keith Dodds – Paediatrician, Derby City General Hospital

The Audit Commission is grateful to them all. Responsibility for the contents and conclusions rests solely with the Audit Commission.

Abbreviations

Abbreviations used in this report

BAPM – British Association for Perinatal Medicine

BPA – British Paediatric Association

CEMD – Confidential Enquiry into Maternal Deaths

CESDI – Confidential Enquiry into Stillbirths and Deaths in Infancy

CSAG – Clinical Standards Advisory Group

FHSA – Family Health Services Authority

HES – Hospital Episode System

MIDIRS – Midwives Information and Resource Service

MSLC – Maternity Services Liaison Committee

NNU – Neonatal Unit

OPCS – Office of Population Censuses and Surveys
(now ONS – Office for National Statistics)

RCM – Royal College of Midwives

RCGP – Royal College of General Practitioners

RCOG – Royal College of Obstetricians and Gynaecologists

RCP – Royal College of Physicians

Glossary

advanced neonatal nurse practitioners
Nurses with specialist training and qualifications. They are able to attend to medical and nursing needs of NNU patients.

antenatal
Before the birth, during pregnancy.

APGAR score
A set of criteria for assessing the well-being of the baby at birth. Scored from 0–10.

artificial rupture of membranes (amniotomy)
Breaking the amniotic sac containing the baby. Usually as a means of beginning or speeding up labour (sometimes along with other methods). Also necessary for some forms of fetal monitoring.

assisted delivery
Delivery of the baby vaginally using forceps or ventouse.

augmentation/acceleration
Speeding labour up artificially with drugs and/or by rupturing the membranes.

booking visit
An antenatal contact during which medical and midwifery services are arranged, including the intended place of delivery and type of care to be provided.

breech presentation
The presentation of the baby bottom or feet first.

caesarean section
Delivery of the baby by cutting through the woman's abdomen and into the womb.

Changing Childbirth
Government maternity policy for England.

Cochrane database
Electronic database of systematic reviews of maternity care.

continuity of care/carer
Continuity of care – care is delivered in a consistent way, regardless of the professional providing it.

Continuity of carer – care is provided by a small number of professionals, or by professionals women know.

DOMINO
'Domiciliary In and Out' – a system in which community midwives visit women in labour at home, escort them into hospital for delivery, and discharge them home following a short (less than 24-hour) hospital stay.

Down's syndrome
A chromosonal disorder. Screening tests to estimate the probability of a baby being affected by Down's syndrome may be offered.

electronic fetal monitoring
Monitoring the baby's heartbeat electronically through a monitor (either externally on a belt around the mother's abdomen, or internally using an electrode attached to the baby's head).

ECV **(external cephalic version)**	A technique for turning breech babies.
epidural analgesia	A local anaesthetic injected into the epidural space around the spinal sac causing loss of sensation to the lower part of the body.
episiotomy	Surgical cut to the perineum to expedite delivery.
forceps delivery	A vaginal delivery using forceps. A form of instrumental delivery.
gestation	Length of pregnancy – usually measured from the last mentrual period.
GP unit	General practitioner maternity unit – a maternity unit in which women book to deliver under the supervision of midwives and GPs. These can be integrated into the main consultant unit, or alongside it, or be completely separate from it.
HELLP Syndrome **(haemolysis, elevated liver enzymes, low platelets)**	A condition associated with eclampsia, a convulsive condition, a serious, potentially life-threatening condition of pregnancy.
in utero	Within the uterus.
induce/induction of labour	Starting labour artificially, using drugs or by rupturing the membranes.
intensive care (neonatal)	Specialist care of newborn babies (up to 28 days old), carried out by specifically trained medical and nursing staff. It may involve assisted ventilation or other specialised procedures.
midwife	A person who is qualified to attend women in uncomplicated pregnancy and childbirth.
MSLC	Maternity Services Liaison Committee. Local committees containing professional and lay representatives from maternity services. Roles vary widely.
neonatal	Referring to the new born (up to 28 days old).
neonatal unit	Hospital departments providing specialist care for babies.
obstetrician	A specialist practitioner in the medical and surgical specialty concerned with pregnancy, delivery and the puerperium, particularly among women with complicated pregnancies.
operative delivery	Delivery by forceps, ventouse or caesarean section.
perinatal	Around the period of birth.
perineum	Area of pelvic floor between vagina and anus.

postnatal Period of time after birth. Usually taken to be up to six weeks after the birth. Midwives' responsibilities continue for at least 10 and up to 28 days after birth.

pre-eclampsia A hypertensive condition of pregnancy causing high blood pressure, protein in the urine and swelling. (This can precede a serious condition called eclampsia – see also HELLP syndrome.)

screening tests The carrying out of test or tests in order to detect abnormalities. In this context screening is undertaken to detect problems in pregnancy (eg, hypertension, proteinuria). Screening tests are also carried out to detect the likelihood of certain fetal abnormalities.

serum screening A screening test carried out on a sample of mother's blood, which when analysed provides an estimate of the probability of the baby being affected by Down's syndrome.

stillbirth A baby which is born dead after 24 completed weeks of pregnancy.

transitional care Special care of babies (who may otherwise require admission to a neonatal unit) usually in a ward close to where mothers are receiving postnatal care. This means that mothers and babies are not separated.

ultrasound scan A procedure which uses sound waves to build up a picture of the baby in the womb.

ventouse delivery or vacuum extraction A form of instrumental delivery in which the baby is delivered vaginally with the aid of a shallow rubber cup fitted to the baby's head using suction.

References

1 House of Commons Health Committee (1992), *Second Report – Maternity Services: Volume 1*, London, HMSO.

2 RCOG, RCM and RCGP (1992), *Maternity Care in the New NHS: A Joint Approach*, Report from Presidents of RCOG and RCM and Chairman of RCGP, London, RCGP.

3 Government Response (1992) to the second report of the health committee: maternity services, Session 1991-92, Cmnd 2018, London, HMSO.

4 Welsh Office (1991), *Protocol for Investment in Health Gain Maternal and Early Child Health*, Welsh Office, Cardiff (protocol currently being updated) and related technical papers.

5 Department of Health (1993), *Changing Childbirth*, Report of the Expert Maternity Group, London, HMSO.

6 Department of Health/Welsh Office 1995, TFR2 *Financial Returns* 1994/95.

7 Kitzinger S et al (1992), Chapter 3 in: Enkin M et al (eds), *A Guide to Effective Care in Pregnancy and Childbirth*, Oxford, OUP.

8 *Report on Confidential Enquiries into Maternal Deaths in the United Kingdom (CEMD) 1991 – 1993*, Department of Health, Welsh Office, Scottish Home and Health Departments, Department of Health and Social Services, Northern Ireland, London, HMSO.

9 *Confidential Enquiry into Stillbirths and Deaths in Infancy (CESDI); Third Annual Report 1 January – 31 December 1994*, London, Department of Health, May 1996.

10 Cochrane Database of Systematic Reviews, *The Cochrane Collaboration, Issue 2*, Oxford, Update Software 1996.

11 Welsh Office (1996), *Maternity Services Review Wales*, Welsh Office, Cardiff.

12 Department of Health, Scottish Office, Welsh Office (1996), *Choice and Opportunity – Primary Care: The Future*, London, Department of Health.

13 Delbanco T (1996), *'Quality of Care Through the Patient's Eyes'*, British *Medical Journal* 313, pp832-3.

14 Brown S et al (1994), *Missing Voices: The Experience of Motherhood*, Oxford, OUP.

15 Oakley A et al (1966), 'Social Support in Pregnancy: Does It Have Long-term Effects?', *Journal of Reproductive and Infant Psychology 14*, pp7-22.

16   Mason V (1989), *Women's Experience of Maternity Care – A Survey Manual*, London, OPCS.

17   Green JM et al (1988), *Great Expectations: A Prospective Study of Women's Expectations and Experiences of Childbirth*, Centre for Family Research, University of Cambridge.

18   Green JM et al (1990), 'Expectations, Experiences, and Psychological Outcomes of Childbirth: A Prospective Study of 825 Women', *Birth 17*, pp15-24.

19   McCourt C and Page L (1996), *Report of the Evaluation of One-To-One Midwifery*. London, Thames Valley University.

20   Smith J et al (1996), 'Debriefing After Childbirth: A Tool for Effective Risk Management', *British Journal of Midwifery* 4 (11), pp581-6.

21   Crompton J (1996), 'Post-traumatic Stress Disorder and Pregnancy'. *British Journal of Midwifery 4 (6)*, pp290-4

22   Maternity Services Advisory Committee (1982), *Maternity Care in Action: A Guide to Good Practice and a Plan for Action*, London, HMSO.

23   Hirst J et al (1996), 'Women's Views of Their First Antenatal Visit', *British Journal of General Practice,* May 1996, p319.

24   Ratcliffe J et al (1996), 'The Costs of Alternative Types of Routine Antenatal Care for Low Risk Women: Shared Care vs Care by General Practitioners and Community Midwives', *Journal of Health Services Research Policy, 1 (3)*, pp135-40.

25   Tucker J et al (1996), 'Should Obstetricians See Women with Normal Pregnancies? A Multicentre Randomised Controlled Trial of Routine Antenatal Care by General Practitioners and Midwives compared with Shared Care led by Obstetricians', *British Medical Journal 312*, pp554-9.

26   Chamberlain G (1994), *The ABC of Antenatal Care*, 2nd edition, London, BMJ Publishing Group.

27   Sikorski J et al (1996), 'A Randomised Controlled Trial Comparing Two Schedules of Antenatal Visits: The Antenatal Care Project', *British Medical Journal 312*, pp 546-53.

28   Munjanja SP et al (1996), 'Randomised Controlled Trial of a Reduced Visits Programme of Antenatal Care in Harare, Zimbabwe', *Lancet 348*, pp364-9.

29   Neilson JP (1996), 'Routine Ultrasound in Early Pregnancy', in Cochrane Database of Systematic Reviews, *The Cochrane Collaboration, Issue 2*, Oxford, Update Software, 1996.

30 Dowswell T et al (1994), 'Antenatal Ultrasound Scanning: Suggestions for Debate', *Midwifery* 10, pp238-43.

31 Santalahti P et al (1996), 'Women's Experiences of Prenatal Serum Screening', *Birth 23* (2), pp101-7.

32 Marteau TM (1995), 'Towards Informed Decisions About Pre-natal Testing: A Review', *Prenatal Diagnosis 15*, pp 1215-26.

33 MIDIRS (1996), Midwives Information and Research Service and NHS Centre for Reviews and Dissemination, *Informed Choice* leaflets, London, MIDIRS.

34 Personal communication. Royal College of Obstetricians and Gynaecologists Audit Unit, St Mary's Hospital, Manchester.

35 Keirse M (1989), 'Social and Psychological Support in Labour', in: *Effective Care in Pregnancy and Childbirth*, (eds Chalmers et al), Oxford, OUP.

36 Hodnett E (1996), 'Support During Childbirth' in Cochrane Database of Systematic Reviews, *The Cochrane Collaboration, Issue 2*, Oxford, Update Sofware.

37 Neilson J (1995), 'EFM and Scalp Sampling vs Intermittent Auscultation in Labour', in Cochrane Database of Systematic Reviews, *The Cochrane Collaboration, Issue 2*, Oxford, Update Software, 1996.

38 Thorp J et al (1996), 'Epidural Analgesia in Labour: An Evaluation of Risks and Benefits', *Birth 23 (2)*, pp63-83.

39 Lomas J et al (1989), 'Variations in Operative Delivery Rates', in *Effective Care in Pregnancy and Childbirth* (eds Chalmers et al), Oxford, OUP.

40 Clinical Standards Advisory Group (1995), *Women in Normal Labour*, London, HMSO.

41 Clark L et al (1991), 'How does Mode of Delivery Affect the Cost of Maternity Care?', *British Journal of Obstetrics and Gynaecology 98*, pp519-23.

42 Drife J (1996), 'Choice and Instrumental Delivery', *British Journal of Obstetrics and Gynaecology 103*, pp608-11.

43 RCOG Audit Committee (1993), *Effective Procedures in Obstetrics Suitable for Audit*, Manchester, RCOG Audit Unit.

44 Enkin M et al (eds) (1992), *A Guide to Effective Care in Pregnancy and Childbirth*, Oxford, OUP.

45 Lomas J (1988), 'Holding Back the Tide of Caesareans', *British Medical Journal* 207, pp569-70.

46 Francome C et al (1993), 'Caesarean Section in Britain and the US – 12 or 24 per cent: Is Either the Right Rate? *Social Science and Medicine 37*, pp1199-218.

47 Mould T et al (1996), 'Women's Involvement with the Decision Preceding Their Caesarean Section and Their Degree of Satisfaction,' *British Journal of Obstetrics and Gynaecology 103*, pp1074-7.

48 Henriksen T (1994), 'Methods and Consequences of Changes in Use of Episiotomy', *British Medical Journal 309*,pp1255-7.

49 Macfarlane A et al (1995), *Counting the Changes in Childbirth: Trends and Gaps in National Statistics*, Oxford, NPEU.

50 RCOG Annual Statistical Return, RCOG, London.

51 Cleary R et al (1996), 'The Standard Primipara as a Basis for Inter-unit Comparisons of Maternity Care', *British Journal of Obstetrics and Gynaecology 103*, pp223-9.

52 Kiwanuka AI and Moore WM (1993), 'Influence of Audit and Feedback on Use of Caesarean Section in a Geographically Defined Population', *European Journal of Obstetrics and Gynaecology and Reproductive Biology 50*, pp59-64.

53 Robson MS et al (1996), 'Using the Medical Audit Cycle to Reduce Caesarean Section Rates', *American Journal of Obstetrics and Gynaecology 174*, pp199-205.

54 Chamberlain G (1993), 'What is the Correct Caesarean Section Rate?', *British Journal of Obstetrics and Gynaecology 100*, pp 403-4.

55 Glazener C et al (1995), 'Postnatal Maternal Morbidity: Extent, Causes, Prevention and Treatment', *British Journal of Obstetrics and Gynaecology 102*, pp282-7.

56 MacArthur C et al (1992), 'Investigation of Long Term Problems after Obstetric Epidural Anaesthesia', *British Medical Journal 304*, pp1279-82.

57 MacArthur C et al (1991), 'Health After Childbirth', (commentary), *British Journal of Obstetrics and Gynaecology 98*, pp1193-204.

58 Bick D and MacArthur C (1995), 'Attendance, Content and Relevance of the Six Week Postnatal Examination', *Midwifery 11*, pp69-73.

59 Sharif K et al (1993), 'Routine Six Weeks Postnatal Vaginal Examination: To Do Or Not To Do', *British Journal of Obstetrics and Gynaecology 13 (4)*, pp251-2.

60 Audit Commission (1992), *Children First*, London, Audit Commission/HMSO.

61 Twaddle S and Harper V (1992), 'An Economic Evaluation of Daycare in the Management of Hypertension in Pregnancy', *British Journal of Obstetrics and Gynaecology 99 (6)*, pp459-63.

62 OPCS (1990), *Infant Feeding 1990*, London, HMSO.

63 BPA (1993), *Neonatal Resuscitation*, Report of a BPA Working Party, BPA, London.

64 Clinical Standards Advisory Group (1993), *Neonatal Intensive Care: Access and Availability of Specialist Services*, London, HMSO.

65 RCP (1988), *Medical Care of the Newborn in England and Wales: A Report by the Royal College of Physicians*, London.

66 Botting B et al (1990), *Three, Four and More: A Study of Triplet and Higher Order Births*, London, HMSO.

67 BAPM (1996), *Standards for Hospitals Providing Neonatal Intensive Care*. London, BAPM.

68 Welsh Office (1989), *Stroud Report: Perinatal Intensive Care Services in Wales*, accompanying DGM (96) 151, Welsh Office, Cardiff.

69 Welsh Office (1996), *Post Implementation Review of Neonatal Intensive Care Services*, Report to the Welsh Office, accompanying letter DGM (96) 151, Welsh Office, Cardiff.

70 Northern and Yorkshire RHA (1995), *Report of Working Party on Neonatal Intensive Care*, Leeds, NYRHA.

71 Field D et al (1991), 'Survival and Place of Treatment After Premature Delivery', *Archives of Disease in Childhood 66*, pp408-11.

72 International Neonatal Network (1993), 'The CRIB (Clinical Risk Index for Babies): A Tool for Assessing Neonatal Risk and Comparing Performance of Neonatal Intensive Care Units', *Lancet 342*, pp193-8.

73 Northern RHA (1992), 3rd report, *Neonatal Services in the Northern Region*, Newcastle, NRHA.

74 Redshaw M et al (1993), 'Nursing and Medical Staffing in Neonatal Units', *Journal of Nursing Management 1*, pp221-8.

75 Redshaw M et al (1996), *Delivering Neonatal Care*, London, HMSO.

76 ENB (1987), *Guidelines for Staffing Neonatal Units*, English National Board (ENB), London.

77 Redshaw M et al (1995), *Breaking New Ground: The Education and Role of the Advanced Neonatal Nurse Practitioner*, London, English National Board for Nursing Midwifery and Health Visiting (ENB).

78 NHS Executive (1993), *Priorities and Planning Guidance*. EL(93)54, Department of Health, Leeds.

79 NHS Executive (1994), *Improving the Effectiveness of the NHS*, EL(94) 74, Department of Health, Leeds.

80 NHS Executive (1994), *Developing NHS Purchasing and GP Fundholding*, EL(94)79, Department of Health, Leeds.

81 NHS Executive (1994), *Woman Centred Maternity Services*, EL (94)9, Department of Health, Leeds.

82 NHS Executive (1996), *Maternity Services Liaison Committees: Guidelines for Working Effectively*, available from the Health Literature Line 0800 555777.

83 Somerset Health Authority (1995), *Somerset Guide to Childbirth*, Taunton, Somerset Health Authority.

84 Paterson-Brown S et al (1993), 'Are Clinicians Interested in Up-to-date Reviews of Effective Care?', *British Medical Journal 307*, p1464.

Bibliography

Baird A et al (1996), 'Management of Labour in an Isolated Rural Maternity Hospital', *British Medical Journal 312*, pp223-6.

Ball J (1992), *Who's Left Holding the Baby*, Leeds, Nuffield Institute for Health Services Research.

Ball J et al (1996), *Birthrate Plus: A Framework for Workforce Planning and Decision-making for Midwifery Service*, Books for Midwives Press.

BAPM Working Group (1989), 'Referrals for Neonatal Medical Care in the UK Over One Year', *British Medical Journal 298*, pp169-72.

BAPM (1992), RWIC/JLM, *Report of the Working Group of the BAPM: Categories of Babies Requiring Neonatal Care*, BAPM/BPA, London.

Bick D and MacArthur C (1994), 'Identifying Morbidity in Post Partum Women', *Modern Midwife* 10-13.

BPA and RCOG Standing Joint Committee (1983), *Midwife and Nurse Staffing and Training for Special Care and Intensive Care of the Newborn*, BPA, RCOG, London.

Campbell R and McFarlane A (1995), *Where To Be Born: The Debate and the Evidence*, Oxford, NPEU.

Dewan G et al (1993), 'Postnatal Pain: A Neglected Area', *British Journal of Midwifery 1 (2)*, pp63-6.

Garcia J (1995), *Continuity of Carer: What Matters to Women?*, Chapter 7 in Page L (eds), *Effective Group Practice in Midwifery*, Basil Blackwell, Oxford.

Glazener C et al (1993), 'Postnatal Care: A Time for Change', *Contemporary Reviews of Obstetrics and Gynaecology 5*, pp130-5.

Glazener C et al (1993), 'Postnatal Care: A Survey of Patients' Experiences', *British Journal of Midwifery 1 (2)*, pp67-74.

Hall M H et al (1980), 'Is Routine Antenatal Care Worthwhile?', *Lancet,* 12 July 1980, pp78-80.

Hodnett E (1993), 'Social Support During High Risk Pregnancy: Does it Help?, *Birth 20*; pp218-9.

Hundley V et al (1994), 'Midwife-managed Delivery Unit: A Randomised Controlled Comparison with Consultant Led Care', *British Medical Journal 309*, pp1400-4.

James DK (1995), 'Obstetricians Should Focus On Problems', *British Medical Journal 310*, pp37-8.

Lilford R (1989), 'Evaluating New Treatments and Diagnostic Technologies', *International Journal of Technology Assessment in Health Care 5*, pp459-73.

Maclean G (1994), 'Safe Motherhood in the UK', *Modern Midwife* 4 (6), pp10-14.

MORI (1993), *Maternity Services Summary Report*, Research Study Conducted for the Department of Health, June 1993.

National Audit Office (1990), *Maternity Services*, London, NAO/HMSO.

Northern Neonatal Network (1993), 'Requirements for Neonatal Cots', *Archives of Disease in Childhood 68*, pp544-9.

Northern Neonatal Network (1993), 'Measuring Neonatal Nurse Workload', *Archives of Disease in Childhood 68*, pp539-43.

Oakley A (1984), *The Captured Womb: A History of Medical Care of Pregnant Women*, Basil Blackwell, Oxford.

O'Brien M and Smith C (1981), 'Women's Views and Experiences of Antenatal Care', *The Practitioner 225*, 123-5.

Pearson V (1994), *Antenatal Ultrasound Scanning, Health Care Evaluation Unit*, University of Bristol.

RCGP (1996), *The Role of General Practice in Maternity Care*, Occasional Paper 72, London, RCGP.

RCOG (1982), *Report of the RCOG Working Party on Antenatal and Intrapartum Care*, London, RCOG.

RCOG (1993), *Report of the RCOG Working Party on Biochemical Markers and the Detection of Down's Syndrome*, London RCOG press.

RCOG (1994), *The Future of Maternity Services*, London, RCOG.

RCOG (1995), *Communication Standards in Obstetrics*, London, RCOG.

RCOG (1995), *Organisational Standards for Maternity Services*, London, RCOG.

Shearer EL (1993), 'Caesarean Section: Medical Benefits and Costs', *Social Science and Medicine* 37 (10), pp1223-31.

Sheldon Report (1971), *Report of the Expert Group on Special Care Babies, DHSS, Report on Public Health and Medical Subjects*, 27, London, HMSO.

Smith DK et al (1994), 'Lack of Knowledge in Health Professionals: A Barrier to Providing Information to Patients?', *Quality in Health Care 3*, pp75-8.

Thornton J et al (1994), 'Active Management of Labour: Current Knowledge and Research Issues', *British Medical Journal* 309, pp366-9.

Tyler S (1996), 'Making GP Fundholding Work for Midwives', *British Journal of Midwifery 4 (8)*, pp431-4.

Williams et al (1993), 'Nursing Requirements for Neonatal Intensive Care', *Archives of Disease in Childhood 68*, pp534-8.

Walker P (1995), 'Obstetricians Should Be Included in Integrated Team Care', *British Medical Journal* 310, pp36-7.

World Health Organisation (WHO) (1985), 'Appropriate Technology for Birth', *Lancet ii*, pp436-7.

Wraight A et al (1993), *Mapping Team Midwifery: A Report to the Department of Health*, IMS Report Series 242, Institute of Manpower Studies, Brighton.

Index
References are to paragraph number, Boxes and Case Studies.

Analgesia   77-9

Antenatal care   20, 25, 38-68

  choices in   40

  community-based   23, 44, 47, 48

  GPs in   43, 45, 46

  hospital-based   20, 40, 42-4, 47

  organisation   42-9

  patterns of   45, 46, *Box D*

  policies   67

  routine tests   60-1

  screening for fetal abnormality   59, 63-8

Antenatal checks

  clinical content   59-68

  number of   53-8

Audit Commission survey of recent mothers   10, Appendix 1, *Box B*

Baby checks   115

Birth

  GP units   72

  home   71, 72

  options   72, 75

Birth companions   76

Breastfeeding   33, 111, 121, 124, 131-4, 154

Caesarean section   92, 94, 99-100, 107, 114, 166

  costs   97

Changing Childbirth   1, 10, 51, 68, 158, 163

Choice   9, 24-7, 35, 45, 72, 78, 100, 105, 163-7

Clinical audit   107, *Case Study 2*

Clinical effectiveness. *See* Effectiveness

Clinical Standards Advisory Group (CSAG)   95

Cochrane database of clinical trials   6, 172-4

Commissioning   66, 157-9, 169, *Case Study 4*

Communication   19, 23, 50, 101, 102, 106, 129, 150, 162-5

Complications in pregnancy   21, 47, 50-2, 58, *Box C*

Continuity of care   9, 28-32, 45

Continuity of carer   28, 29, 31, 36, 51, 57, 90-1

Contracts, maternity services   158

Costs   2, 45, 49, 65, 84, 97, 127, 170

Data – maternity   34, 56, 103, 104, 133, 134, 140, 156, 169, 171

Debriefing facility   27, 129

Delivery rooms   76, 80-3

Education and training   58, 91, 106

Effectiveness   6, 7, 9, 37, 47, 69, 92-107, 111, 124, 157, 171-6

Efficiency   7, 9, 37, 58, 100, 114-27, 167, 168-70, 175

Emotional support   17, 69, 79

Epidural analgesia   76, 78, 79

Episiotomy   26, 74, 101

Evidence-based practice   172-3

  see also effectiveness

Forceps delivery   92, 98

Fragmentation of service delivery   9, 28,160-2

GP maternity care   9, 42, 43, 45, 46, 157, 159, 161-2

Home birth   71, 72

Home visits   110

  postnatal   124-7, *Case Study 3*

Hospital Episode System (HES)   103

Hospital facilities

  labour   70, 80-3

  postnatal care   128-30

Infant feeding   131-4, 154

Information provision   9, 13, 16, 19, 23, 26, 33-5, 40, 50, 51, 58, 62, 64, 65, 68, 79, 100-2, 105, 152, 162-7

Instrumental deliveries   92, 96, 98, 106

Labour   21, 26, 33, 69

  continuity of carer   29, 90-1

  decisions to induce or accelerate   74

  options   70

  professional support during   84-5

  staffing levels   84-91

Labour wards   70, 76

  facilities   80-3

  staff organisation   86-9

Length of stay - postnatal   27, 114-19

Litigation   99, 100

Maternity Services Liaison Committees (MSLCs)   34, 157

Medical interventions   5, 92-107

Medical staffing, neonatal
units (NNUs)   146-9

Midwives

   organisation   30, 71, 81, 86-9, 120

   antenatal care   42-6

   labour   71, 84, 91

   postnatal care   120-3

Midwives Information and
Resource Services (MIDIRS)   68, 164

Neonatal units (NNUs)   108, 120,
                              123, 135-54

   activity   138-42

   admission rates   139

   medical cover   146-9

   parental support   150-4

   planning   140-1

   staffing   143-9

Obstetricians   5, 6, 42, 43, 45,
                            46, 65, 92-107, 158,
                                      166-7

Paediatricians   5, 6, 115, 116,
                           123, 138, 139, 142,
                                  146, 149

Pain relief   77-9

Policy   7, 156, *Box A*

Postnatal care   110, 112

   efficient   114-27

   home visits   22, 31, 124-7,
                               Case Study 3

   hospital-based   22, 27, 31, 110, 112

   hospital facilities   128-30

   length of hospital stay   27, 114-19

   quality of   22, 31, 112, 119,
                            121, 128-34, 138

   staffing   120-3

Postnatal check   111

Postnatal health problems   96, 109, 126

Pre-eclampsia   60-1, 92

Professional support during
labour   84-5

Safety   15, 69, 128

Scans   25, 63-8

Screening tests   25, 59-68

Social support   50, 69

Specialist services   50-2

Staffing levels   33

   labour wards   84-91

   neonatal units (NNUs)   143-9

   postnatal   120-3

Standard primipara   104

Stitches   101

Team/caseload midwifery   30, 86, 88,
                               120, 122

Tears   101

Transitional care wards   138

Ultrasound scanning   25, 63-8

Variations in patterns of care   156-9

Ventouse delivery   92, 98, 106

Welsh Office   7, 55, *Box A*

   see also policy

Woman-centred care   7, 15, 33, 57,
                             163-7, *Box A*

Women's perceptions
and attitudes   8, 14, 16-22, 31,
                            33, 37, 75, 84,
                           102, 112, 117,
                               118, 130